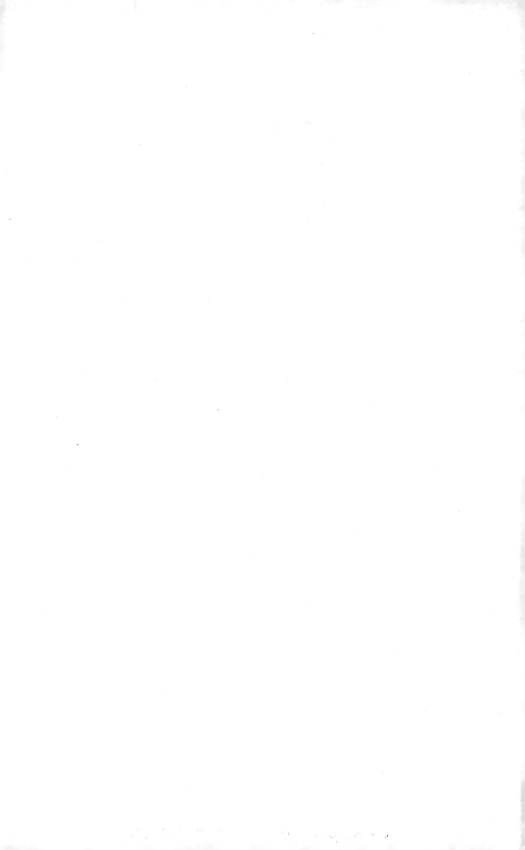

LOCAL ANESTHETICS

Mechanisms of Action
and Clinical Use

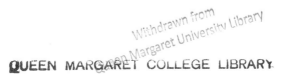

THE SCIENTIFIC BASIS OF CLINICAL ANESTHESIA

Series Editors

RICHARD J. KITZ, M.D.
MYRON B. LAVER, M.D.

Other Books in the Series

ANESTHESIA AND THE KIDNEY
   R. Dennis Bastron, M.D. and Stanley Deutsch, Ph.D., M.D.

LOCAL ANESTHETICS

Mechanisms of Action and Clinical Use

Benjamin G. Covino, Ph.D., M.D.

Scientific Director
Research and Development Division
Astra Pharmaceutical Products, Inc.
Framingham, Massachusetts

Professor of Anesthesiology
University of Massachusetts
Worcester, Massachusetts

Helen G. Vassallo, Ph.D.

Head, Data Evaluation
Department of Clinical Trials
Research and Development Division
Astra Pharmaceutical Products, Inc.
Framingham, Massachusetts

GRUNE & STRATTON
A Subsidiary of Harcourt Brace Jovanovich, Publishers
New York   London
Paris   San Diego   San Francisco   São Paulo
Sydney   Tokyo   Toronto

Library of Congress Cataloging in Publication Data

Covino, Benjamin G

   Local anesthetics.

   (Scientific basis of clinical anesthesia)
   Includes bibliographical references and index.
   1. Local   anesthesia. I.   Vassallo,   Helen   G.,   joint   author.   II.   Title.
[DNLM: 1.   Anesthetics, Local—Phamacodynamics.   QV110 C873L]
RD84.C68   617'.966   75-35749
ISBN 0-8089-0918-5

Grune & Stratton, Inc.
111 Fifth Avenue
New York, New York 10003

Distributed in the United Kingdom by
Academic Press, Inc. (London) Ltd.
24/28 Oval Road, London NW1

Library of Congress Catalog Card Number 75-35749
International Standard Book Number 0-8089-0918-5
Printed in the United States of America

Dedicated to
Lorraine, Paul and Brian

Contents

Introduction

As this series begins it is time to ask ourselves several questions. Is the practice of anesthesia exclusively art rather than science? Has the specialty achieved a level of sophistication where at least a part of the anesthesia experience has a rational explanation? Have we reached that stage when new concepts and understanding are evolving from within the specialty at a rate adequate to assure growth and permanence? We have good reason to believe we are approaching the latter evolutionary phase and are bending to retrieve the gauntlet cast in 1950 by William T. Salter, M.D., Professor of Pharmacology at Yale. In "The Leaven of the Profession" (Anesthesiology 11:374–376, 1950) he wrote:

"At this juncture, however, those who have the future of Anesthesiology close at heart will realize that no professional specialty can maintain itself on the basis of service alone. In the case of Surgery, for example, Harvey Cushing—one of the most skilled technicians of his day—once intimated that it might be well if amputation of the fingers were a requirement for an appointment to the Chair of Surgery in every progressive university." This remark annoyed quite a few of the contemporary super-technicians whom Cushing counted among his colleagues! Nevertheless, his remark contained a very important germ of truth; namely, that professions do not live by service alone, but rather by the words of wisdom which issue out of the mouths of those few demigods who in every generation lead and inspire the multitude of their professional associates.

"In this day and age there is a tendency for the routine anesthetist to 'pass the buck' to the professor of physiology or the professor of pharmacology, in the vain hope that the answers can be learned from mice or monkeys. The respective professors named are usually only too eager to cooperate and interested in fostering the development of applied studies on man. They realize all too well, however, that such studies must be made by an applied pharmacologist, appointed by the Department of Anesthesiology. Such a man should be familiar with the everyday problems of the practicing Anesthesiologist. He should have basic training in the fundamental departments mentioned. He would do well perhaps to commence his work with experiments on animals performed under the aegis of the pre-clinical departments. Ultimately, however, the problem must be taken into the clinic and the definitive answers resolved there.

"To this end, there must be trained a group of so-called 'academic Anesthesiologists.' These individuals must have the special training and sufficient leisure to advance the basic concepts of applied science. In their earlier years they must be supported by adequate fellowships. In their mature years they must receive adequate recognition in the form of staff appointments and university affiliation. They must not be run ragged with routine assignments, but must be protected from the irate surgeon who demands service now in the name of all humanity and the Trustees. At the present time the fellowships and funds available for this purpose are pitifully meager. . . . The conscientious and overworked anesthetist, while rendering invaluable service to the community, fails to appreciate that his ultimate professional status cannot be guaranteed by service alone. Without vision and research, the professions die."

It is the intention of the editors to provide the specialty with a monograph series targeted to the clinical areas. In the Salter tradition, the authors are clinicians, distinquished additionally by their contributions to the scientific base of our specialty. Superb clinicians who simultaneously function as dedicated investigators are a rare hybrid able to filter effectively the relevant signals from laboratory noise and transduce the data into comprehensible and applicable information. The editors are especially proud to have secured the services of a distinguished faculty for this pupose.

We accept the tenet that the informed practitioner who roots his clinical decisions in a nidus of relevant science is bound to render superior patient care. It is to that end that we dedicate the Scientific Basis of Clinical Anesthesia.

Richard J. Kitz, M.D.
Myron B. Laver, M.D.

Boston, 1976

Acknowledgments

The authors wish to acknowledge the efforts of those people whose assistance made this monograph possible: Mrs. Betty French who typed and retyped the many drafts without complaint, Mrs. Joyce Serafin whose artistic abilities made possible the numerous tables and illustrations, and the entire staff of the research and development division of the Astra Company who provided much of the unpublished data presented in this monograph.

LOCAL ANESTHETICS

Mechanisms of Action
and Clinical Use

1

Chemical Aspects of Local Anesthetic Agents

HISTORICAL NOTES

Local anesthesia may be defined as a loss of sensation in a circumscribed area of the body due to a depression of excitation in nerve endings or an inhibition of the conduction process in peripheral nervous tissue. This localized state of anesthesia may be produced by such different means as mechanical trauma, low temperature, anoxia, and a variety of chemical irritants. In general, only substances that produce a transient and completely reversible state of insensibility are employed in clinical practice. Neurolytic agents such as alcohol or phenol may be useful to induce a relatively permanent state of anesthesia in patients with intractable pain.

The use of chemical substances to prevent or treat local pain had its origin in South America during the nineteenth century. It was known that central nervous system stimulation occurred among the natives of Peru who chewed the leaves of an indigenous plant (*Erythroxylon coca*). Circumoral numbness was believed to have occurred as a by-product of this custom. Attempts to isolate the active principle from leaves of the *Erythroxylon coca* bush resulted in the extraction of the alkaloid, erythroxylon, by Gaedcke in 1855 and finally in the isolation of the alkaloid, cocaine, by Niemann in 1860.[1] The potential use of cocaine as a local anesthetic agent was initially described by a Peruvian army surgeon, Moréno y Maïz, in an obscure monograph.[2] However, the clinical usefulness of cocaine was not appreciated until 1884, when Koller reported that instillation of cocaine into the conjunctival sac resulted in topical anesthesia of the eye.[3] These observations led to the widespread use of cocaine as a topical anesthetic agent in ophthalmology. Within a year after Koller's discovery of the topical anesthetic properties of cocaine, Halstead administered this substance by injection for the production of peripheral nerve blockade. By 1898, spinal anesthesia with cocaine had been performed by Bier. These early experiments represented a major advance in surgery. However, a number of adverse effects, both acute and chronic, were observed with the clinical use of cocaine. The acute effects were due to systemic toxicity and the chronic effects were due to cocaine's addicting properties. The severity of these adverse reactions resulted in an intense effort to develop chemical substances possessing the beneficial local anesthetic properties of cocaine, but without such serious side effects. One of the major programs in the present field of local anesthesia is to develop local anesthetic drugs with a more favorable therapeutic ratio.

The chemical identification of cocaine as a benzoic acid ester led to the synthesis of numerous compounds which were basically benzoic acid ester derivatives. Benzocaine, a poorly water-soluble local anesthetic agent, was identified by Ritsert in 1890.[4] Because its low water solubility limited its usefulness as an injectable agent, this compound was neglected for many years. Ultimately, benzocaine was recognized as an effective topical anesthetic agent and persists today as a valuable drug for the production of surface anesthesia of mucous membranes. In 1905, Einhorn and Braun reported the synthesis of procaine, an ester of para-aminobenzoic acid.[5, 6] Procaine was water soluble, fairly stable in solution, and possessed an acceptable margin of local and systemic safety for clinical use as an injectable agent in regional anesthesia.

Following the introduction of procaine, numerous similar compounds were synthesized. Tetracaine, the most potent ester of the benzoic acid series appeared in 1930[7] and chloroprocaine, the least toxic of this chemical group, was initially described in 1952.[8] These two para-aminobenzoic acid derivatives are still widely used clinically as local anesthetic agents.

Until the mid-twentieth century, most compounds synthesized as local anesthetic agents were, like tetracaine and chloroprocaine, benzoic acid derivatives. Unfortunately, the major drawback to this chemical class of substances has been their propensity for producing allergic or sensitizing-type reactions. A major breakthrough in the chemistry of local anesthetic agents occurred in 1943 when Löfgren synthesized lidocaine.[9] Lidocaine represented a major chemical de-

Table 1

REPRESENTATIVE LOCAL ANESTHETIC AGENTS IN COMMON CLINICAL USE

Generic* and Common Proprietary Name	Chemical Structure	Approx. year of Initial Clinical Use	Main Anesthetic Utility	Representative Commercial Preparation
Cocaine	$CH_2-CH-CHCOOCH_3$ / $NCH_3-CHOOC_6H_5$ / $CH_2-CH-CH_2$	1884	Topical	bulk powder
Benzocaine / Americaine*	$H_2N-C_6H_4-\overset{O}{C}-OC_2H_5$	1900	Topical	20% ointment 20% aerosol
Procaine / Novocain*	$H_2N-C_6H_4-COOCH_2CH_2N(C_2H_5)_2$	1905	Infiltration Spinal	10 and 20 mg/ml solutions 100 mg/ml solution
Dibucaine / Nupercaine*	quinoline ring $-OC_4H_9$ $CONHCH_2N(C_2H_5)_2$	1929	Spinal	0.667, 2.5 and 5 mg/ml solutions
Tetracaine / Pontocaine*	H_9C_4 $\overset{H}{N}-C_6H_4-COOCH_2CH_2N(CH_3)_2$	1930	Spinal	Niphanoid crystals - 20 mg/ml 10 mg/ml solutions
Lidocaine / Xylocaine*	$C_6H_3(CH_3)_2-NHCOCH_2N(C_2H_5)_2$	1944	Infiltration Peripheral Nerve Blockade Epidural Spinal Topical "	5 and 10 mg/ml solutions 10, 15 and 20 mg/ml sol'ns 10, 15 and 20 mg/ml sol'ns 50 mg/ml solution 2.0% jelly, viscous 2.5%, 5.0% ointment
Chloroprocaine / Nesacaine*	$H_2N-C_6H_3(Cl)-COOCH_2CH_2N(C_2H_5)_2$	1955	Infiltration Peripheral Nerve Blockade Epidural	10 mg/ml solution 10 and 20 mg/ml solutions 20 and 30 mg/ml solutions
Mepivacaine / Carbocaine*	$C_6H_3(CH_3)_2-NHCO-$ piperidine $-CH_3$	1957	Infiltration Peripheral Nerve Blockade Epidural	10 mg/ml solution 10 and 20 mg/ml solutions 10, 15 and 20 mg/ml solutions
Prilocaine / Citanest*	$C_6H_3(CH_3)_2-NHCOCH-NH-C_3H_7$ / CH_3	1960	Infiltration Peripheral Nerve Blockade Epidural	10 and 20 mg/ml solutions 10, 20 and 30 mg/ml solutions 10, 20 and 30 mg/ml solutions
Bupivacaine / Marcaine*	$C_6H_3(CH_3)_2-NHCO-$ piperidine $-C_4H_9$	1963	Infiltration Peripheral Nerve Blockade Epidural	2.5 mg/ml solutions 2.5 and 5 mg/ml solutions 2.5, 5 and 7.5 mg/ml solutions
Etidocaine / Duranest*	$C_6H_3(CH_3)_2-NHCOCHN(C_2H_5)$ / C_3H_7	1972	Infiltration Peripheral Nerve Blockade Epidural	2.5 and 5 mg/ml solutions 5 and 10 mg/ml solutions 5 and 10 mg/ml solutions

*USP nomenclature

parture from the previous local anesthetic drugs, since it was not an ester but an amide derivative of diethylamino acetic acid. Not only did this new class of amide-type local anesthetic agent offer certain advantages in terms of anesthetic activity, but more importantly, perhaps, such compounds appeared to be relatively free of the sensitizing reactions characteristic of the ester-type derivatives of para-aminobenzoic acid. Since the advent of lidocaine, all newer local anesthetic agents introduced into clinical practice have been essentially amide-type structures. Thus, mepivacaine, prilocaine, bupivacaine, and etidocaine, which represent the most recent additions to the local anesthetic armamentarium, are amide-type chemical compounds similar to lidocaine, that differ somewhat in their pharmacological profile from lidocaine and from each other.

Representative local anesthetic agents presently in common clinical use are listed in Table 1. The generic name, trade name, and chemical structure of each of these compounds are presented, in addition to their main anesthetic utility and the various types of available commercial preparations.

CHEMICAL CLASSIFICATION OF
LOCAL ANESTHETIC AGENTS

Blockade of nerve conduction can be produced by a great variety of chemical structures. Substances that can be classified in broad terms as amino-esters, amino-carbamates, amino-ketones, amidines, alcohols, thioesters, thioethers, thioamides, ureas, phosphoric esters, polyethers, and simple amines are capable of impeding the conduction process in isolated or intact nerves.[10] In general, those local anesthetic agents of proven clinical utility have been the amino-esters and amino-amides.

Amino-Esters

As mentioned previously, most of the agents in this category are ester derivatives of para-aminobenzoic acid. Benzocaine (ethyl 4-aminobenzoate), the oldest of the currently available ester-type agents, is still used widely as a topical anesthetic agent, particularly in nonprescription preparations recommended for dermal pain from minor abrasions or sunburn. Procaine (2-diethylaminoethyl 4-aminobenzoate) was for many years the standard injectable local anesthetic agent for use in infiltration, peripheral nerve blockade, and central neural blockade. Procaine possesses poor topical anesthetic properties and its current clinical role is limited essentially to infiltration procedures. Other similar compounds that still enjoy wide clinical utility are tetracaine and chloroprocaine. Tetracaine (2-dimethylaminoethyl 4-butylaminobenzoate), most potent of the amino-ester agents in clinical use, is employed as both an injectable and a topical analgesic compound. Tetracaine still remains the most commonly used drug for spinal anesthesia. Chloroprocaine (2-diethylaminoethyl 4-amino-2-chlorobenzoate), the least toxic agent in this class, is particularly suitable for short surgical procedures in poor-risk patients. The structures of benzocaine, procaine, tetracaine, and chloroprocaine are presented in Table 1.

Amino-Amides

Lidocaine (2-diethylaminoacet-2, 6-xylidide), which was the first compound in this series of chemical structures to demonstrate clinical utility as a local anesthetic agent, represented such a significant pharmacological advance over procaine that it soon replaced procaine as the standard local anesthetic drug. Chemically related amide compounds have been introduced into clinical practice during recent years. Prilocaine (2-propylamino-2'-propionotoluidide) differs chemically from lidocaine in that it is a toluidine derivative and secondary amine, whereas lidocaine is a xylidine derivative and tertiary amine.[11] The main clinical advantage of this agent is its relatively low systemic toxicity. Etidocaine (2-N-ethylpropylamino-2',6'-butyroxylidide), the most recent local anesthetic agent introduced into clinical practice, also is structurally similar to lidocaine, but possesses a greater anesthetic potency and a longer duration of action.[12]

Ekenstam, Egner, and Pettersson described a series of amino-amides in which the chain amino group was made part of a ring system by joining one of the aminoalkyl groups with the intermediate acyl chain.[13] Mepivacaine (1-methyl-2',6'-hexahydropicolinylxylidide) was the initial compound in this series to be introduced into clinical practice.[14] This agent has properties similar to those of lidocaine but lacks topical anesthetic qualities. Bupivacaine (1-butyl-2',6'-hexahydropicolinylxylidide), a homologue of mepivacaine, possesses a greater anesthetic potency and prolonged duration of action compared to mepivacaine.[15]

Guanidine-Type Structures

A third category of substances possessing potent local anesthetic activity includes the guanidine-type molecules. Tetrodotoxin and saxitoxin, representatives of this group, appear in Figure 1-1.[16, 17] Tetrodotoxin is derived from the ovaries and other organs of the puffer fish found most commonly along the coast of Japan.[18] Saxitoxin is produced by certain marine dinoflagellates which can contami-

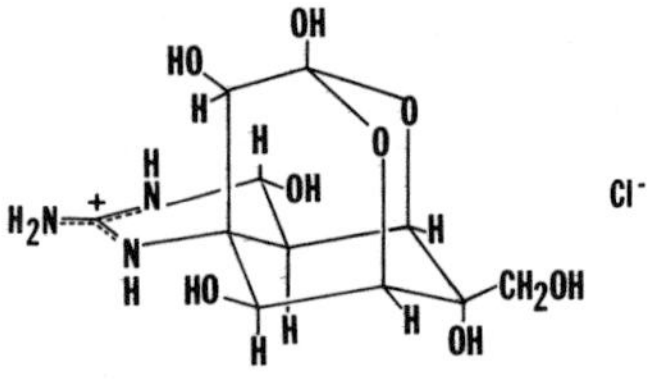

TETRODOTOXIN

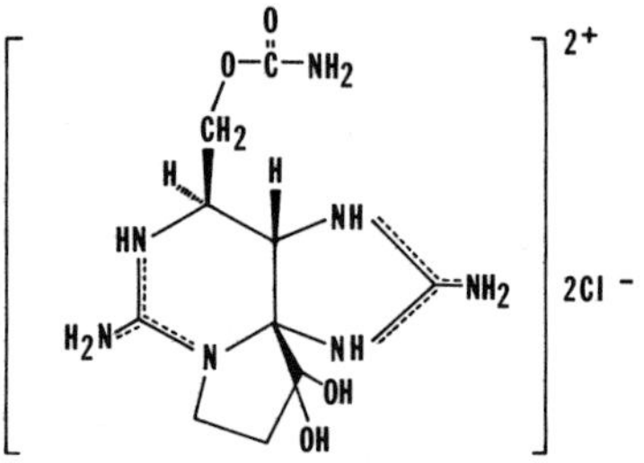

SAXITOXIN

Fig. 1-1. Chemical structures of tetrodotoxin as described by Goto et al.[16] and saxitoxin as suggested by Schantz et al.[17]

nate shellfish and cause paralytic shellfish poisoning in man.[19] Both of these biotoxins are quite different chemically from other types of local anesthetic agents, since they contain guanidine moieties, resulting in compounds that are stronger bases than either the amino-esters or amino-amides. These substances are the most potent inhibitors of nerve conduction studied to date. Although not presently available for clinical use, such compounds as tetrodotoxin and saxitoxin may be of importance in the future. A classification of these chemical substances according to their biological site of action will be presented in a later chapter.

STRUCTURE-ACTIVITY RELATIONSHIPS

As indicated above, a great variety of chemical structures may produce conduction blockade in nerves. Therefore, it is difficult to define precisely the relationship between the chemical structure and biological activity of local anesthetic agents. However, compounds that demonstrate clinical utility as local anesthetic agents, in general, possess the following chemical arrangement:

Aromatic Portion—Intermediate Chain—Amine Portion

The aromatic portion of the molecule is believed responsible for the lipophilic properties, whereas the amine end is associated with hydrophilicity. Alterations in the aromatic portion, amine portion, or intermediate chain of a specific chemical compound will modify its anesthetic activity. For example, an increase in molecular weight within an homologous series of compounds, achieved by lengthening the intermediate chain or by the addition of carbon atoms to either the aromatic or amine portion of the molecule, will tend to increase intrinsic anesthetic potency up to a maximum, beyond which a further increase in molecular weight results in a decrease in anesthetic activity.[10] Changes in the aromatic or amine portion of a local anesthetic substance will alter its lipid/water distribution coefficient and its protein-binding characteristics which, in turn, will markedly alter the anesthetic profile within a series of homologous compounds. The relationship between chemical structure, partition coefficient, protein-binding, and anesthetic activity of various homologous anesthetic agents is presented in Table 2. A comparison between procaine and tetracaine, which are both ester derivatives of para-aminobenzoic acid, reveals that the addition of a butyl group to the aromatic end of the procaine molecule produces a greater than 100-fold increase in lipid solubility and a ten-fold increase in protein-binding.[20] Such changes in physicochemical properties are reflected in marked alterations in biological activity. For example, the intrinsic anesthetic potency of tetracaine as determined on an isolated nerve is approximately 16 times greater than that of procaine, whereas the duration of its anesthetic activity as determined in vivo in the rat sciatic nerve preparation is approximately four times longer than that of procaine.

Similar relationships exist in the amide series of compounds. The addition of a butyl group to the amine end of mepivacaine, forming bupivacaine, results in a 35-fold increase in partition coefficient[21] and a significantly greater degree of protein-binding as compared to mepivacaine. The chemical alterations of mepivacaine to bupivacaine and the subsequent modification of physicochemical properties result in a four-fold increase in intrinsic anesthetic activity and a significant prolongation of anesthetic duration.

Another example of the relationship between modification of chemical structure and biological activity is found in the comparison of lidocaine and etidocaine. Substitution in the lidocaine molecule of a propyl for an ethyl group at the amine end and the addition of an ethyl

Table 2

STRUCTURE - ACTIVITY RELATIONSHIP OF LOCAL ANESTHETIC AGENTS

AGENT	CHEMICAL CONFIGURATION			PHYSICO-CHEMICAL PROPERTIES		BIOLOGICAL PROPERTIES		
	Aromatic Lipophilic	Intermediate Chain	Amine Hydrophilic	Partition Coefficient	% Protein Binding	Equi-Effective* Anesthetic Conc.	Approx. Anesthetic* Duration (min)	Site of Metabolism
A. Esters PROCAINE	H_2N-⟨⟩	COOCH$_2$CH$_2$	$-N\begin{smallmatrix}C_2H_5\\C_2H_5\end{smallmatrix}$	0.6[1]	5.8[3]	2	50	Plasma
TETRACAINE	$\begin{smallmatrix}H_9C_4\\H\end{smallmatrix}N-$⟨⟩	COOCH$_2$CH$_2$	$-N\begin{smallmatrix}CH_3\\CH_3\end{smallmatrix}$	80[1]	75.6[3]	0.25	175	Plasma
B. Amides MEPIVACAINE	⟨⟩$\begin{smallmatrix}CH_3\\CH_3\end{smallmatrix}$	NHCO	CH$_3$ N⟨⟩	0.8[2]	77.5[4]	1	100	Liver
BUPIVACAINE	⟨⟩$\begin{smallmatrix}CH_3\\CH_3\end{smallmatrix}$	NHCO	C$_4$H$_9$ N⟨⟩	27.5[2]	95.6[4]	0.25	175	Liver
LIDOCAINE	⟨⟩$\begin{smallmatrix}CH_3\\CH_3\end{smallmatrix}$	NHCOCH$_2$	$-N\begin{smallmatrix}C_2H_5\\C_2H_5\end{smallmatrix}$	2.9[2]	64.3[4]	1	100	Liver
ETIDOCAINE	⟨⟩$\begin{smallmatrix}CH_3\\CH_3\end{smallmatrix}$	NHCOCH C$_2$H$_5$	$-N\begin{smallmatrix}C_2H_5\\C_3H_7\end{smallmatrix}$	141[2]	94[4]	0.25	200	Liver

[1] oleylalcohol / pH 7.2 buffer   [3] nerve homogenate binding   *data derived from rat sciatic nerve blocking procedure
[2] n-heptane/ pH 7.4 buffer   [4] plasma protein binding - 2μg/ml

group at the alpha carbon in the intermediate chain yields etidocaine. These chemical changes in structure produce an increase in partition coefficient of approximately 50-fold and a significant increase in protein-binding.[22] As in the previous examples, these alterations in chemical structure and physicochemical properties are reflected in significant changes in biological activity, such that etidocaine possesses an intrinsic anesthetic potency four times greater than that of lidocaine and a duration of anesthetic action approximately twice that of lidocaine.

The rate of degradation and subsequently intrinsic toxicity also will be affected by alterations in the chemical structure of homologous compounds. A comparison of the three ester local anesthetic agents—i.e., tetracaine, procaine, and chloroprocaine—reveals a considerable difference in the rate of enzymatic hydrolysis and intrinsic toxicity of these three agents (Table 3). Tetracaine, which is hydrolyzed quite slowly, shows an LD$_{50}$ value of 48 mg/kg following

Table 3

RELATIONSHIP BETWEEN THE RATE OF HYDROLYSIS AND SUBCUTANEOUS TOXICITY OF
SEVERAL ESTER- TYPE LOCAL ANESTHETIC AGENTS

Agent	Rate of Hydrolysis (μ moles/ml/hr)	Subcutaneous Toxicity in mice (LD_{50} values)	Main Products of Metabolism
CHLOROPROCAINE	4.7	1,396	2 chloro,4-aminobenzoic acid, diethylaminoethanol
PROCAINE	1.1	615	4-aminobenzoic acid, diethylaminoethanol
TETRACAINE	0.3	48	4-butylaminobenzoic acid, diethylaminoethanol

subcutaneous administration in mice,[23] whereas chloroprocaine, which undergoes rapid hydrolysis, has an LD_{50} value of 1396 mg/kg in mice. Procaine is intermediate between chloroprocaine and tetracaine, both in terms of rate of hydrolysis and intrinsic toxicity (LD_{50} value of 615 mg/kg). A similar relationship exists within the amide series between lidocaine and prilocaine. Prilocaine is metabolized at a significantly more rapid rate by liver enzymes than is lidocaine and possesses an intrinsic toxicity significantly less than that of lidocaine.[24] A further comparison of prilocaine and lidocaine reveals an interesting aspect of structure-activity relations. The presence of methyl groups in the 2,6-position of the benzene ring of lidocaine results in the formation of 2,6-xylidine as one of the metabolites of lidocaine. On the other hand, prilocaine, lacking the methyl group in the 6-position of the benzene ring has as one of its primary metabolites, o-toluidine. The formation of o-toluidine can induce the production of methemoglobin and is responsible for the methemoglobinemia observed clinically in patients receiving high doses of prilocaine.[25] Lidocaine administration does not result in the formation of methemoglobin.

Alterations in chemical structure within an homologous series of local anesthetic agents are reflected in changes in intrinsic anesthetic potency, duration of action, rate of degradation, and intrinsic toxicity. The basic differences between heterologous local anesthetic agents, i.e., the ester and amide compounds, are: (a) the manner in which they are metabolized and (b) their allergic potential. The ester derivatives of benzoic acid are hydrolyzed primarily in plasma by the enzyme pseudocholinesterase.[26] Members of the amide series of local anesthetic compounds undergo enzymatic degradation primarily in the liver.[27, 28] The difference in site of metabolism between these two main classes of local anesthetic agents is of clinical relevance. Patients possessing a genetic deficiency in the enzyme, pseudocholinesterase, are unable to hydrolyze these drugs at a normal rate and show reduced tolerance to ester-type local anesthetic agents. Moreover, pseudocholinesterase is responsible for the degradation of neuromuscular blocking agents of the depolarizing types such as succinylcholine. The concomitant use of neuromuscular blocking agents such as succinylcholine and ester-type local anesthetic agents may result in a prolonged duration of neuromuscular blockade and increased toxicity of the local anesthetic agent.[29] Use of a local anesthetic agent of the amide-type in such clinical situations is preferable, since these agents do not depend on the enzyme, pseudocholinesterase, for their metabolism. On the other hand, patients with liver disease may show reduced tolerance to the amide-type local anesthetic drugs, since they are metabolized mainly by hepatic microsomal enzymes. In such patients, the normal dose of an amide agent should be reduced or a compound of the ester-type substituted.

Since the ester agents are derivatives of para-aminobenzoic acid, this substance occurs as a metabolite following hydrolysis of the parent compound. This metabolite is responsible for the allergic-type reactions observed in a small percentage of the general population exposed to such agents. The amide lidocaine-like drugs are not metabolized to para-aminobenzoic acid and reports of allergic phenomena with this group of agents are extremely rare. No evidence of cross sensitivity between the amino-esters and amino-amides has been reported.

SUMMARY

1. Isolation of cocaine from the *Erythroxylon coca* bush marked the start of the local anesthetic era in clinical medicine.
2. The clinically useful drugs presently available essentially fall into two chemical categories: (a) agents with an ester link between the aromatic end of the molecule and the intermediate chain (procaine-like); (b) agents with an amide link between the aromatic portion and the intermediate group (lidocaine-like).
3. Chemical alterations within an homologous group produce quantitative changes in: (a) physicochemical properties, i.e., lipid solubility and protein-binding, which, in turn, alter the anesthetic profile of the compounds; (b) rate of metabolism and type of metabolites formed, which affect systemic toxicity in a quantitative and qualitative fashion.
4. The chemical difference between heterologous groups is reflected

biologically in (a) site of metabolism, i.e., ester compounds are hydrolyzed in plasma whereas amide compounds undergo enzymatic degradation in the liver, and (b) allergic potential, i.e., a greater frequency of sensitizing reactions is observed with the ester derivatives of para-aminobenzoic acid.

2

Pharmacodynamic Aspects
of Local Anesthetic Agents

ANATOMY OF PERIPHERAL NERVE

Peripheral nerves are mixed nerves containing both sensory afferent fibers and motor efferent fibers. Figure 2-1 presents a cross-sectional view of a typical peripheral nerve and illustrates some of the anatomical factors that influence the pharmacological properties of local anesthetic agents. Peripheral nerves possess a distinctive organizational pattern. Each individual axon is surrounded by a connective tissue sheath known as the endoneurium. Groups of axons are enclosed in an additional connective tissue sheath called the perineurium. Finally, a number of axonal groups are encased in an external connective tissue sheath, the epineurium. Interference with the conduction process by pharmacological means requires diffusion of chemical compounds through these connective tissue layers to the individual axonal fiber. Thus, the epineurium, perineurium, and endoneurium are considered anatomical barriers to the diffusion of local anesthetic substances. Differences exist with regard to the rate at which various local anesthetic agents diffuse through these connective tissue sheaths. The physicochemical properties of individual compounds themselves and the physiological state of the local milieu surrounding the nerve fibers will determine the rate of diffusion and ultimately the onset of analgesia.

A consideration of the morphological features of the axon itself also reveals certain barriers that may influence the movement of local anesthetic agents. Figure 2-2 presents a diagrammatical cross-sectional sketch of a myelinated and unmyelinated nerve. An un-

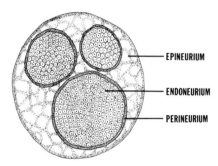

Fig. 2-1.   Cross-sectional diagram of a peripheral nerve.

myelinated nerve fiber is surrounded by a single wrapping, the Schwann cell sheath. Groups of unmyelinated fibers share the same Schwann cell. All postganglionic fibers of the autonomic nervous system and fibers less than 1 micron in diameter (C fibers) in the somatic nervous system are unmyelinated, e.g., pain fibers and motor fibers to involuntary muscles.

Myelinated fibers are enclosed in spirally wrapped layers of lipoprotein myelin sheaths which are actually a specialized form of a Schwann cell. Each myelinated fiber is enclosed in its own myelin sheath. The outermost layer of myelin essentially consists of the Schwann cell cytoplasm and its nucleus. The myelin sheath surround-

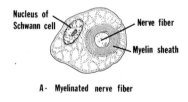

A- Myelinated nerve fiber

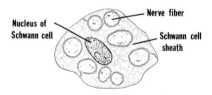

B- Un-myelinated nerve fibers

Fig. 2-2.   Comparative morphology of myelinated and unmyelinated nerves.

ing a myelinated nerve fiber (A & B fibers) is interrupted at intervals by constrictions, i.e., the nodes of Ranvier. The size of the individual Schwann cell determines the distance between adjacent nodes. These myelin sheaths are essentially lipid in nature (75%), but also contain some protein (20%) and carbohydrate (5%) material.[30] The molecular structure of these myelin sheaths has been described by various investigators as consisting of two bimolecular leaflets of lipid with polar heads pointing outward and each polar surface covered by a monolayer of protein.[31-33] However, the precise molecular configuration of this lipoprotein membrane is still a matter of some debate.

In addition to the connective tissue and myelin, or Schwann cell sheath, enveloping nerve fibers, the neuronal axon possesses its own cell membrane, the axolemma, which surrounds the axoplasm. Various molecular structures have been proposed for biological membranes including the axonal membrane. Danielli and Davson originally suggested that the cell membrane consisted of a lipid core arranged in such a fashion that the polar lipid heads were oriented in an outward direction and were covered by a nonlipid monolayer which was probably protein in nature.[34] Several modifications of this basic model have been proposed.[35-37] In 1959, Robertson advocated the term "the unit membrane" as the fundamental unit of all biological membranes.[33, 36] The unit membrane was visualized as consisting of a bimolecular leaflet of unspecified lipids at the center with the polar lipid heads pointed outward and covered on both exposed surfaces by a monolayer of nonlipids. This model differed from that of Danielli and Davson in that the nonlipid layers covering the internal and external surface of the polar lipid heads were believed to differ in chemical composition. Although the exact structure and chemical composition of the unit membrane may not be accepted universally, it is generally believed that biological membranes do consist essentially of a lipoprotein matrix arranged in a fashion somewhat similar to that shown in Figure 2-3.

More recent membrane models visualize proteins rather than lipids as the basic organizational elements of membranes.[38-40] Although the importance of lipids as an essential part of the membrane is still appreciated, current models describe the membrane as being heterogenous in nature with a greater interaction between protein and lipid molecules such as shown in Figure 2-4. A comparison of various models depicting the molecular structure of the cell membrane is presented in Figure 2-5.[41]

Although the axolemma was known to consist mainly of lipids and to a lesser degree protein and carbohydrates, the exact composi-

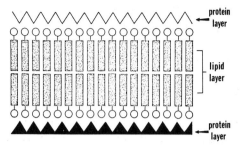

Fig. 2-3.   Unit membrane as suggested by Robertson.[36]

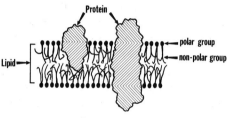

Fig. 2-4.   Heterogeneous   lipoprotein   membrane   as
suggested by Singer.[40]

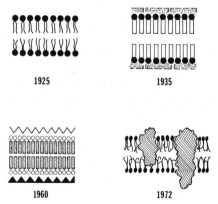

Fig. 2-5.   Comparison of various cell membrane models
suggested between 1925 and 1972.

tion was not well known. The most complete chemical analysis of the axolemma was accomplished by Camejo and co-workers in 1969.[42] Utilizing the first stellar nerve of the giant squid, these authors extruded the axoplasm and subjected the remaining material to centrifugation. Two fractions were obtained in this manner. That fraction possessing the greater enzymatic activity was assumed to be the axolemma and contained both proteins and lipids. The protein to lipid ratio for the squid axolemma was 0.13, indicating that the greatest portion (almost 90%) of the axolemma consisted of lipids, mainly, phospholipids such as phosphatidyl choline, phosphatidyl ethanol amine, phosphatidyl serine, and sphingomyelin (Table 4).

Irrespective of the precise structure and composition of the nerve membrane, it is apparent that lipids and proteins play an essential role in the molecular organization of these membranes. This suggests that the physicochemical properties of local anesthetic agents, namely lipid solubility and protein-binding, are important in terms of the ultimate interaction between specific local anesthetic drugs and the nerve membrane. This interrelationship between the physicochemical properties of specific agents, the structure of the nerve membrane, and the resultant biological action, can be demonstrated if one compares certain homologous local anesthetic compounds. For example, lidocaine and etidocaine are related amide-type local anesthetic agents that possess similar pK_a values, but differ markedly in their lipid solubility and protein-binding characteristics. A comparison of the biological effect of these two agents on the isolated frog sciatic nerve reveals that etidocaine has a more rapid onset of conduction

Table 4

PERCENTAGE WEIGHT COMPOSITION OF MEMBRANE
FRACTIONS ISOLATED FROM GIANT SQUID NERVE

PROTEIN	29.5 ± 1.4
TOTAL LIPIDS	70.5 ± 1.5
CHOLESTEROL	28.1 ± 2.3
FATTY ACIDS	6.2 ± 0.9
POLAR LIPIDS	58.5 ± 3.5
PHOSPHATIDYL CHOLINE	45.9 ± 2.9
SPHINGOMYELIN	10.0 ± 1.6
PHOSPHATIDYL ETHANOLAMINE	34.4 ± 1.7
PHOSPHATIDYL SERINE	10.4 ± 2.3

Data derived from Camejo et al (1969)

blockade, a greater potency, and a longer duration of action.[43] These biological effects are consistent with the greater lipid solubility of etidocaine, which suggests that it should diffuse through the lipid myelin sheath and axonal membrane more easily and so have a shorter latency. The greater protein-binding capacity implies that it should bind to a greater degree with the protein component of the membrane and, thus, be an agent of greater intrinsic anesthetic potency and longer duration of action (Fig. 2-6). The basic relationship

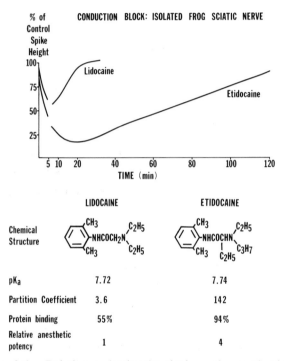

Fig. 2-6. Relative physicochemical and conduction-blocking properties of lidocaine and etidocaine.

between nerve morphology, chemical structure, and physicochemical properties of local anesthetic compounds may be obscured under clinical conditions due to other biological factors. However, ulnar nerve block studies in man, comparing lidocaine and etidocaine, reveal results similar to those obtained on the isolated frog sciatic nerve, which suggest that these fundamental anatomical-chemical-biological interrelations can be demonstrated clinically (Fig. 2-7). [44]

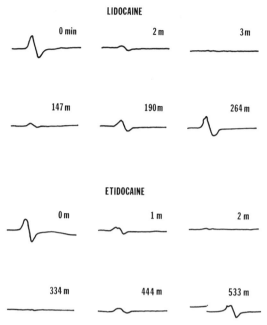

Fig. 2-7. Hypothenar electromyographs prior to and following ulnar nerve block with 1% lidocaine and 0.5% etidocaine.

PHYSIOLOGY OF PERIPHERAL NERVE

Membrane Electrophysiology

Local anesthetic agents exert their primary pharmacological action by interfering with the excitation-conduction process of peripheral nerve fibers and nerve endings. The development of microelectrodes that could be inserted intracellularly has made possible biophysical studies that have provided information concerning the basic electrophysiological properties of nerve tissue.[45] Figure 2-8 graphically depicts the transmembrane action potential of the peripheral nerve as recorded by such an intracellular electrode.[44]

During the period of nerve inactivity, a negative electrical potential (resting potential) of approximately -60 to -90 mv exists across the cell membrane. When excitation occurs, a consistent sequence of events takes place. An initial phase of depolarization is observed during which the electrical potential within the nerve cell becomes

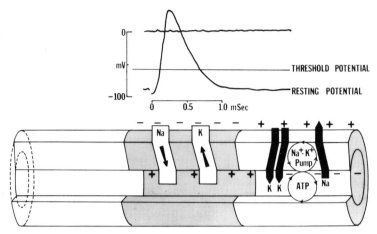

Fig. 2-8.   Relationship between membrane action potential and ionic flux across the nerve membrane.

progressively less negative. When the potential difference between the interior and exterior surface of the cell membrane reaches a critical level, the threshold potential, or firing level, an extremely rapid phase of depolarization commences which results in a reversal of the electrical potential across the cell membrane, such that the inside of the membrane becomes positively charged with respect to the outside of the cell membrane. At the peak of the action potential, the interior of the cell has a positive electrical potential of approximately $+40$ mv as compared to the exterior of the cell. After completion of the depolarization phase, repolarization begins, and during this time, the electrical potential within the cell again becomes progressively more negative with respect to the exterior of the cell until such time as the resting potential of -60 to -90 mv is reestablished. Under normal conditions, this entire process of depolarization and repolarization occurs within 1 msec. The depolarization phase occupies approximately 30% of the entire action potential whereas repolarization accounts for the remaining 70%.

Membrane Electrochemistry

The electrophysiological properties of the nerve membrane are dependent on (a) the concentration of electrolytes in nerve cytoplasm and extracellular fluid and (b) the permeability of the cell membrane to various ions—particularly, sodium and potassium. The ionic composition of the cytoplasm and the extracellular fluid differ markedly.

The intracellular concentration of potassium is approximately 110 to 170 meq/1, whereas the intracellular concentration of sodium and chloride ions is approximately 5–10 meq/l. In extracellular fluid, the situation is reversed. The concentration of sodium is approximately 140 meq/l and the concentration of chloride is 110 meq/l, whereas the extracellular concentration of potassium is 3–5 meq/l.

This ionic asymmetry on either side of the cell membrane is due in part to the selective permeability characteristics of the membrane. The resting membrane is fully permeable to potassium ions, but only slightly permeable to sodium ions, which accounts for the low intracellular concentration of sodium. The high intracellular concentration of potassium is maintained by the attractive forces of the negative charges, mainly on proteins, within the cell which counterbalances the tendency of potassium ions to diffuse out of the cell by passive movement along a concentration gradient and across a freely permeable membrane. Nernst derived an equation to predict the electrical potential across a membrane separating two concentrations of the same ion:

$$E = -\frac{RT}{nF} \ln \frac{[A]_i}{[A]_o}$$

E = membrane potential between inside and outside of the cell
R = gas constant in joules (8.315)
T = absolute temperature
n = valence of the ion
F = Faraday's constant (96,500 coulombs)
ln = natural logarithm

At room temperature (18°C) and assuming a K_i/K_o ratio across the nerve membrane of 30, i.e., $[150 \text{ meq/l}]_i/[5 \text{ meq/l}]_o$, the Nernst equation would predict the following:

$$E = -58 \log \frac{[30K]_i}{[K]_o}$$

$$E = -85.7 \text{ mv}$$

This predicted resting membrane potential of -85.7 mv agrees closely with the commonly reported values of -60 to -90 mv measured directly in nerve preparations with intracellular electrodes. Thus, at rest, the nerve cell behaves as a potassium electrode that would react to intra- or extracellular changes in potassium concentrations, but not sodium concentrations. Indeed, the resting membrane potential of nerves can be altered by changes in the potassium content of extracellular fluid, but is unaffected by variations in the sodium concentration.[46]

Attempts have been made to utilize clinically the relationship between the resting potential and the K_i/K_o ratio. Thus, potassium chloride has been added to solutions of local anesthetic agents in an attempt to combine the conduction blocking effects of a reduced resting potential and an anesthetic drug. The duration of action and quality of anesthesia produced by procaine can be increased by the concomitant use of KCl in a concentration of 135–150 mM.[47] The addition of KCl to solutions of lidocaine has been reported to decrease the onset time and improve the quality of epidural anesthesia[48] and to prolong the duration of digital and ulnar nerve blocks in man.[49]

Membrane Activation

Excitation of a nerve results in an increase in the permeability of the cell membrane to sodium ions. The initial flux of sodium ions from the exterior of the cell membrane to the interior of the nerve cell results in a depolarization of the cell membrane from the resting potential level to the threshold or firing level of approximately −50 to −60 mv. At this point, a maximum increase in the permeability of the cell membrane to sodium ions occurs and an explosively rapid influx of sodium ions into the axoplasm follows. At the end of depolarization or at the peak of the action potential, the nerve membrane is essentially transformed from a potassium electrode to a sodium electrode and the positive membrane potential of +40 mv can be calculated again from the Nernst equation by substituting the ratio of sodium ions between the inside and outside of the nerve membrane (Na_i/Na_o) for the potassium ion ratio (K_i/K_o).

At the conclusion of the depolarization phase, the permeability of the cell membrane to sodium ions again decreases and high K^+ permeability is restored. Potassium moves out of the cell, resulting in repolarization of the membrane until such time as the original electrochemical equilibrium and resting potential is reachieved. The flux of sodium ions into the cell during depolarization and potassium ions out of the cell during repolarization is a passive phenomenon, since each ion is moving down its concentration gradient.

The relationship of the membrane potential to the potassium and sodium permeabilities and gradients can be described by an extension of the basic Nernst equation:[50, 51]

$$E = -\frac{RT}{nF} \ln \frac{P_K[K]_i + P_{Na}[Na]_i + P_{Cl}[Cl]_o}{P_K[K]_o + P_{Na}[Na]_o + P_{Cl}[Cl]_i}$$

If the permeability of one ion species is markedly greater than any other, the concentration gradient of that particular ion will predict the membrane potential. Following excitation of a nerve cell, the level of the membrane potential at any point in time during the depolarization and repolarization process will be a function of the relative permeabilities and gradients of the various ions.

Following return of the membrane to the resting potential level, a very slight excess of sodium ions is present within the cell and a very slight excess of potassium ions exists outside of the nerve cell. Although the excitation process has been completed and the nerve cell is electrically quiescent, a metabolically active period commences. Restoration of the normal ionic gradient across the nerve membrane requires the expenditure of energy for the active transport of sodium ions from the inside to the outside of the nerve cell against a concentration gradient. This active transport of sodium ions is made possible by the function of the so-called sodium pump. The energy required to drive the sodium pump is derived from the oxidative metabolism of adenosine triphosphate. It has been shown that dinitrophenol, which interferes with oxidative phosphorylation, can prevent the active transport of sodium from the nerve cell, which suggests that the sodium pump is dependent on phosphorylation mechanisms.[52] Addition of excess adenosine triphosphate to a dinitrophenol-treated axon can reverse the inhibition of sodium efflux and restore the rate of sodium extrusion to normal. This metabolic pump, which actively extrudes intracellular sodium ions, also is believed responsible, in part, for the transport of potassium ions from the extracellular space to the interior of the nerve cell, since potassium ions also must move against a concentration gradient in order to restore the normal K_i/K_o ratio across the cell membrane. Potassium will return to the interior of the cell until the electrostatic attraction of the intracellular negative charges balances the chemical concentration gradient.

MECHANISM OF ACTION OF LOCAL ANESTHETIC AGENTS

Electrophysiological Actions

On the basis of the electrophysiological properties of peripheral nerve, it is conceivable that local anesthetic agents could interfere with the excitation process in nerve membrane in one or more of the following ways: alteration of the basic resting potential of the nerve membrane; alteration of the threshold potential or firing level; decrease in the rate of depolarization; and prolongation of the rate of

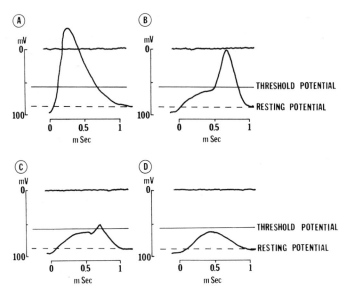

Fig. 2-9. Effect of 0.2 m*M* lidocaine on nerve membrane action potential.
Panel A is a control recording. Panels B, C, and D represent recordings
following exposure to lidocaine.

repolarization. Figure 2-9 shows the changes in the transmembrane
action potential which occur following immersion of an isolated nerve
in a local anesthetic solution. No alteration in the membrane resting
potential of isolated nerves has been observed following exposure to
varying concentrations of different local anesthetic agents such as
procaine or lidocaine.[53, 54] In addition, little or no change in the
threshold potential or firing level occurs following application of local
anesthetic agents to an isolated nerve. Thus, these compounds do not
impede the excitation process in nerve by altering either the resting
potential   or   threshold   potential.   The   predominant   electrophysiological alteration occurs during the depolarization phase of
the action potential. Studies by Aceves and Machne have shown a
decrease in the maximum rate of rise of the action potential of the
isolated lumbar spinal ganglion of the frog from a control value of 190
v/sec to 120 v/sec after 15 minutes exposure to a solution of 0.005%
(0.2 m*M*) lidocaine.[54] This marked decrease in the rate of the depolarization phase, particularly the phase of slow depolarization, is
not accompanied by any significant change in the rate of repolarization. In summary, the primary electrophysiological effect of local
anesthetic agents on the nerve membrane involves a reduction in the

rate of rise of the depolarization phase of the action potential. When cellular depolarization is not sufficient to reduce the membrane potential of the individual fiber to the firing, or threshold potential, a propagated action potential fails to develop.

Effect on Ionic Flux

Since the depolarization phase of the action potential is associated with an influx of sodium ions from the extracellular to intracellular space and since the primary electrophysiological effect of local anesthetic agents involves the depolarization phase of the action potential, it appears logical that local anesthetic agents probably interfere with sodium permeability. Condouris evaluated the interrelationship between sodium ions and cocaine on the surface action potential of the isolated frog sciatic-peroneal nerve trunk.[55] A series of dose-response curves relating concentration of cocaine and the height of the spike potential were determined in Ringer's solution containing various concentrations of sodium. As the concentration of sodium in the bathing solution was decreased, substantially less cocaine was required to reduce the height of the spike potential. As shown in Figure 2-10, at a normal sodium concentration of 116 mmoles, approximately 3.2 mmoles of cocaine were required to produce a 50% decrease in the height of the spike potential. When the sodium concentration was lowered to 12 mmoles, only 0.15 mmoles of cocaine

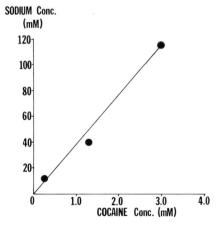

Fig. 2-10.   Relationship between sodium and cocaine concentration required to produce a 50% decrease in nerve-surface action potential.

were necessary to cause a similar reduction in the amplitude of the spike potential. These data suggest that a competitive antagonism exists between local anesthetic agents and sodium with regard to depolarization of the nerve cell.

Direct measurements of sodium and potassium conductance have been carried out utilizing voltage clamp techniques[56-61] to demonstrate that local anesthetic agents block sodium currents in nerve. For example, Hille used the isolated frog sciatic nerve, in which the membrane potential was held at the normal resting potential of -75 mv and demonstrated that 1 mmole of lidocaine produced a complete loss of sodium current.[57] This effect was attributable to a reduction of sodium conductance by lidocaine. At the same time, 3.5 mmoles of lidocaine caused only a 5% decrease in potassium conductance. Therefore, although a decrease in permeability of the cell membrane to potassium can be observed when high local anesthetic concentrations are applied to isolated nerve, this reduction in potassium permeability is considerably less than the decrease in sodium permeability produced by significantly lower concentrations of the local anesthetic agents. These data agree with electrophysiological studies, which show primarily a decrease in the rate of depolarization following exposure of isolated nerves to local anesthetic drugs and only a slight prolongation of repolarization. Additional evidence that the reduction of potassium currents is not an essential component of conduction blockade by local anesthetic agents was obtained in studies in which tetraethylammonium and tetrodotoxin were utilized. Potassium conductance can be blocked completely by tetraethylammonium in frog-myelinated nerve fibers without any accompanying inhibition of the action potential.[62] On the other hand, tetrodotoxin, the puffer fish poison, causes complete inhibition of sodium conductance and complete blockade of the action potential of isolated nerves at a concentration of 30 nM without any discernible effect on potassium conductance.[57] These data indicate that the primary action of local anesthetic agents involves: (a) a reduction in the permeability of the cell membrane to sodium ions; (b) subsequent decrease in the rate of rise of the depolarization phase of the action potential; and (c) failure of a propagated action potential to develop, which ultimately causes conduction blockade.

Calcium-Local Anesthetic Interaction

Calcium ions, which are known to exist in the membrane in a bound state, may exert a regulatory role on the movement of sodium ions across the nerve membrane. The release of bound calcium has been suggested as the primary factor responsible for the increase in the sodium permeability of the nerve membrane and, thus, may represent the initial step in the depolarization process.[63] Therefore, inhibition of sodium conductance by local anesthetic agents may be due, in part at least, to a local anesthetic-calcium interaction.[64-66] Electrophysiological studies by Aceves and Machne have examined the interrelationship of calcium and local anesthetic drugs.[54] Addition of procaine to the bathing solution surrounding an isolated nerve in the presence of a normal concentration of calcium produces a marked decrease in the rate of depolarization and the amplitude of the action potential and an inhibition of a propagated action potential. However, if the calcium concentration is increased from a normal value of 1.8 mmoles to 18 mmoles, the rate of depolarization and the height of the spike potential return to their control values despite the continued presence of the local anesthetic agent in the bathing solution, and ultimately a propagated action potential can be made to reappear. The reversal of the depressant effect of procaine on the rate of depolarization and amplitude of the isolated nerve action potential by an increase in the calcium concentration is demonstrated in Figure 2-11.

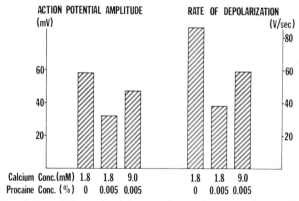

Fig. 2-11.   Effect of calcium and procaine on action potential amplitude and rate of depolarization of isolated nerve.

In the absence of a local anesthetic agent, an increased calcium concentration alone produces inconsistent effects on the spike potential amplitude and actually decreases slightly the rate of depolarization.[54]

These results indicated that the local anesthetic molecules might compete with calcium for some site on the nerve membrane. Additional support for this hypothesis was forthcoming from the studies by Kuperman, Altura, and Chezar, in which isolated frog sciatic nerves were immersed in Ringer's solution containing labeled calcium (^{45}Ca) for 8 hours.[67] The nerves were then placed in calcium-free Ringer's solution and the rate of calcium efflux from nerve to the bathing solution was determined. Addition of 20 mmoles procaine to the nerve bath markedly accelerated the rate of efflux of radioactive calcium from the isolated nerve. A similar increase in calcium release by procaine was obtained in an isolated sartorius muscle preparation. In addition, a comparison of tetracaine and procaine revealed that 5 mmoles of tetracaine produces a 100% greater increase in rate of calcium efflux from sartorius muscle than 50 mmoles of procaine, which suggests a correlation between the anesthetic potency of procaine and tetracaine and their ability to displace calcium from the membrane.

Finally, an interrelationship has been demonstrated between calcium, local anesthetic agents, and sodium flux. Direct measurements of sodium conductance by voltage clamp techniques have shown that the local anesthetic inhibition of sodium conductance can be reversed by increasing the calcium ion concentration.[58, 68] Conversely, reduction in calcium concentration accentuates the inhibitory effect of local anesthetic drugs on sodium conductance. Moreover, saxitoxin binds specifically to the sodium channels in nerve membranes and calcium ions are capable of displacing saxitoxin from this binding site.[69]

Under normal physiological conditions, calcium is probably bound to the phospholipids which constitute the major portion of the lipid element in the cell membrane. Displacement of calcium from this phospholipid-binding site may represent the initial step in the increased permeability of the membrane to sodium ions that ultimately results in membrane depolarization. Blaustein and Goldman have studied the effect of various local anesthetic agents on the binding of calcium to an in vitro phospholipid model and have correlated this action with the local anesthetic activity of the compounds.[59] A reasonable correlation existed between the ability of these agents to suppress the surface action potential of the isolated frog sciatic nerve and their ability to inhibit calcium binding to phosphatidyl-L-serine (Fig. 2-12). For example, lidocaine was found to be 3.5 times as potent as procaine in terms of inhibiting the binding of calcium to phosphatidyl-L-serine and 3.8 times as potent as procaine in blocking conduction in the isolated frog sciatic nerve. Although the above studies clearly indicate an interaction between calcium and local anesthetics, most authorities doubt that calcium plays an essential role in the pro-

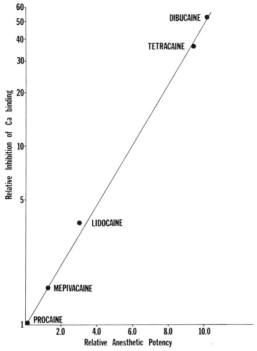

Fig. 2-12.   Relationship of inhibition of calcium binding to anesthetic potency.

duction of local anesthesia. The following sequence is generally accepted as the mode of action of local anesthetic agents: a) reduction in permeability of the cell membrane to sodium ions; (b) decrease in the rate of depolarization of the membrane action potential; (c) lack of development of a propagated action potential; and (e) conduction blockade.

ACTIVE FORM OF LOCAL ANESTHETIC AGENTS

Most of the clinically useful local anesthetic preparations are available in the form of solutions of a salt. For example, lidocaine is usually prepared as an 0.5 to 2.0% aqueous solution of lidocaine hydrochloride. In solution, the salts of these local anesthetic compounds exist both in the form of uncharged molecules (B) and as positively charged cations (BH^+). The relative proportion between

Table 5

SEQUENCE OF EVENTS OF LOCAL ANESTHETIC BLOCK

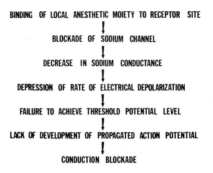

BINDING OF LOCAL ANESTHETIC MOIETY TO RECEPTOR SITE

BLOCKADE OF SODIUM CHANNEL

DECREASE IN SODIUM CONDUCTANCE

DEPRESSION OF RATE OF ELECTRICAL DEPOLARIZATION

FAILURE TO ACHIEVE THRESHOLD POTENTIAL LEVEL

LACK OF DEVELOPMENT OF PROPAGATED ACTION POTENTIAL

CONDUCTION BLOCKADE

the uncharged base (B) and the charged cation (BH^+) depends on the pH of the solution and on the pK_a of the specific chemical compound. The relation between these various factors can be expressed simply as follows:

$$pH = pK_a - \log (BH^+ - B)$$

The total concentration of the local anesthetic agent (C) in solution or at the site of injection is equal to the amount present in the cationic form and the amount present as base.

$$C = BH^+ + B$$

Since the pK_a is constant for any specific compound, the relative proportion of free base and charged cation in the local anesthetic solution depends essentially on the pH of the solution ($BH^+ \rightleftharpoons B + H^+$). Thus, knowledge of the pK_a of a specific compound, the pH of the solution, and the total concentration of the local anesthetic agent would make it possible to determine the relative amounts of the compound that are present in the cationic and base form. As the pH of the solution is decreased and the hydrogen ion concentration is increased, the equilibrium will shift toward the charged cationic form and, thus, relatively more cation will be present than free base. Conversely, as the pH is increased and hydrogen ion concentration decreased, the equilibrium will be shifted toward the free base form, and relatively more of the local anesthetic agent will exist in the free base form rather than as the charged cation.

Much of the early work carried out on isolated intact peripheral nerves indicated that local anesthetic agents were more efficacious when prepared as alkaline solutions. Since more of the uncharged base (B) is present in alkaline solutions, these results suggest that the uncharged base form of the local anesthetic moiety was responsible for the actual anesthetic activity.[70] However, these earlier studies probably failed to take into account that two factors are involved in the ultimate anesthetic action of a chemical compound, i.e., diffusion through the nerve sheath and binding at the receptor site in the cell membrane. To evaluate the difference between diffusion through the nerve sheath and binding at a receptor site, Ritchie, Ritchie, and Greengard carried out a series of studies evaluating the interrelation between the pH of solutions of lidocaine and dibucaine, presence or absence of the nerve sheath, and local anesthetic activity.[71, 72] These investigators used both an isolated frog sciatic nerve and an isolated rabbit vagus nerve preparation. When isolated nerves possessing an intact sheath were studied, it was found that as the pH of the bathing solution containing either lidocaine or dibucaine was raised from 7.2 to 9.2, the rate of reduction in the height of the surface action potential was markedly increased. Thus, alkaline solutions containing relatively greater amounts of the uncharged base (B) were more active in suppressing electrical activity of the sheathed nerve preparations. This observation was consistent with those previously reported by earlier investigators. However, when the experiment was repeated with the use of a desheathed frog sciatic nerve or rabbit vagus nerve preparation, the results differed. Under these experimental conditions, a less alkaline local anesthetic solution, which would result in the formation of a relatively greater amount of the charged cation (BH^+), increased local anesthetic activity. On the basis of these observations, Ritchie, Ritchie, and Greengard postulated that both the uncharged base form (B) and the charged cationic form (BH^+) of local anesthetic agents are involved in the total process of penetration and conduction block. The uncharged base form is believed responsible for optimal diffusion through the nerve sheath. After penetration of the sheath, re-equilibrium occurs between the base and cationic form, and, at the cell membrane itself, the charged cation binds to the receptor site and is ultimately responsible for suppression of the electrophysiological events observed in peripheral nerve[73] (Fig. 2-13). Additional evidence supporting the cationic form of local anesthetic agents as the active moiety was forthcoming from studies in which quaternary ammonium analogues of lidocaine were employed.[74, 75] These compounds, which can only exist in the form of charged cations and not as uncharged bases, were found to be as

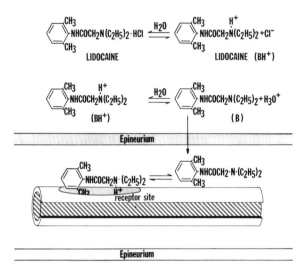

Fig. 2-13.   Diffusion of base form of local anesthetic agent
across epineurium and subsequent binding of cationic form
with receptor site at nerve membrane.

active in blockade of conduction in peripheral nerves as their tertiary
amine analogues. Furthermore, Catchlove has studied the permeability
of isolated nerve sheaths to local anesthetic agents and has reported
that the permeability of these agents is a linear function of the fraction
of nonionized drug present in solution.[76]

Knowledge that the cationic form of local anesthetic agents is
mainly responsible for the conduction blocking action of this class of
compounds has definite clinical relevance. It has been known for
many years that carbon dioxide can potentiate some of the actions of
local anesthetic agents.[77] Catchlove has reported that CO_2 potentiation of local anesthetic activity is due, at least in part, to the increased
formation of the active cationic form by lowering the pH at the nerve
membrane where the local anesthetic receptor is believed to reside.
Catchlove demonstrated that continuous equilibration of Ringer's
solution containing local anesthetic agents with 9.6% carbon dioxide
resulted in a significantly greater suppression of the height of the
nerve action potential than achieved by either procaine, lidocaine, or
bupivacaine without CO_2.[78] For example, 1 mmole bupivacaine reduced the height of the surface action potential of the isolated frog
sciatic nerve to 62% of control value. Equilibration with 9.6% carbon
dioxide and bupivacaine reduced the height of the surface action
potential to 6% of the control value within 5 minutes. The role of the

Table 6

EFFECT OF CO_2 ON THE ANESTHETIC PROPERTIES OF LIDOCAINE AND PRILOCAINE
IN EPIDURAL ANESTHESIA

	Onset Time Mean ± S.D.	Time to Complete Spread	Sensory Duration	Average Degree of Motor Block
2.0 % LIDOCAINE HCl	5.5 ± 1.1	16.0 ± 2.6	97 ± 19.0	36.3%
1.75% LIDOCAINE CO_2	3.6 ± 0.9	10.6 ± 1.6	108 ± 12.8	51.5%
2.0 % PRILOCAINE HCl	7.3 ± 1.8	17.3 ± 2.4	97 ± 10.5	36.3%
1.71% PRILOCAINE CO_2	4.1 ± 1.0	13.1 ± 2.1	113 ± 16.7	48.3%

cationic form of local anesthetic agents in this CO_2 potentiation was substantiated by the inability of carbon dioxide to potentiate the action of N-butanol, a nonionizable local anesthetic compound. Clinical studies have been conducted in which carbonated solutions of lidocaine and prilocaine have been employed for epidural anesthesia and brachial plexus blockade.[79-81] Bromage and co-workers have reported a significant decrease in the onset of epidural anesthesia and an improvement in the quality of epidural anesthesia with the carbonated solutions of lidocaine and prilocaine[79, 80] (Table 6). Similarly, a faster onset of sensory anesthesia following brachial plexus blockade has been reported when solutions of lidocaine equilibrated with CO_2 were employed.[81]

SITE OF ACTION OF LOCAL ANESTHETIC AGENTS

Electrophysiological and biochemical studies have clearly implicated the nerve membrane as the site at which local anesthetic agents exert their pharmacological action. Cellular metabolism of nerves is not inhibited by local anesthetic compounds employed in therapeutic concentrations.[82, 83] Although metabolic inhibitors are capable of producing conduction blockade, the nature of the block is considerably different from that caused by local anesthetic agents.[84] Adenosine triphosphate (ATP), which is intimately involved in reestablishment of the sodium-potassium gradient across the nerve membrane by way of the so-called sodium-potassium pump, has been reported to prevent and reverse conduction blockade by procaine in the isolated frog sciatic nerve.[85] This effect of ATP may be suggestive of a metabolic inhibitory effect of local anesthetic agents, which indirectly cause a decrease in sodium conductance. However, this antagonism between ATP and procaine was not shown to be competitive in nature, since an increase in procaine concentration was not able to overcome the ATP antagonism. Moreover, conduction blockade due to an impairment of the sodium pump by an inhibitory effect on ATP should have been accompanied by a change in the membrane resting potential. As indicated previously, local anesthetic activity is not associated with a change in the resting membrane potential. Although the explanation for the ATP-procaine interaction is not clear, ATP inhibition is not believed responsible for the conduction blocking properties of local anesthetic drugs. In addition, these agents have been found to have no effect on the electrogenic component of the sodium pump in nerves.[86]

Membrane Receptor

The interaction between sodium ions, calcium ions, and local anesthetic agents is suggestive of a specific receptor site for local anesthetic agents at the nerve membrane. Two types of studies have been conducted to support the concept of a membrane receptor for local anesthetic agents. In vitro biochemical investigations have revealed that local anesthetic agents can bind to isolated proteins and phospholipids, which suggests that receptor binding sites for local anesthetic compounds could exist in the membrane.[87] Additional evidence supporting the presence of specific local anesthetic receptors is derived from studies in which optical isomers of local anesthetic agents have been separated and their relative ability to impede neural conduction evaluated.[88,89] Akerman has conducted a detailed investigation of the anesthetic properties of such optical isomers and has observed as much as a fivefold difference in intrinsic anesthetic potency between optical isomers of certain specific local anesthetic agents.[90, 91] These data have been interpreted as suggestive of specific steric requirements for the interaction of a local anesthetic drug and a receptor site in the excitable nerve membrane.

The exact location of a local anesthetic receptor in the nerve membrane also has been the subject of considerable investigation. Hille and co-workers[92] and Strichartz[93] have presented data which suggest that this local anesthetic receptor is probably located at or near the sodium channel in the nerve membrane. Futhermore, it has been postulated that receptors may be present either on the external surface of the sodium channel or on the internal axoplasmic surface of the sodium channel. Local anesthetic compounds have been classified according to their ability to react with receptor sites on either the external or internal portion of the sodium channel.

EXTERNAL RECEPTOR SITE

Only the two biotoxin substances, tetrodotoxin and saxitoxin, have been clearly demonstrated as inhibiting sodium conductance by an effect on the external surface of the sodium channel. Narahashi, Anderson, and Moore have perfused the giant squid axon both externally and internally with solutions of tetrodotoxin.[94] External perfusion with $1 \times 10^{-7}M$ tetrodotoxin prevented the development of a propagated action potential within 3–6 minutes. On the other hand, internal perfusion with $1 \times 10^{-6}M$ and $1 \times 10^{-5}M$ tetrodotoxin for 17–37 minutes had no effect on any component of the action potential. These data suggest that tetrodotoxin inhibits the movement of sodium ions by an interaction with receptor sites on the external surface of the nerve membrane.

INTERNAL RECEPTOR SITE

Certain quaternary ammonium compounds, structurally similar to clinically useful local anesthetic agents such as lidocaine have been found to block conduction when applied to the internal surface of the nerve membrane.[74] Application of these compounds to the external surface of the nerve membrane results in either no conduction blockade or an extremely slow development of block. For example, Strichartz has reported that sodium currents in single myelinated fibers obtained from the sciatic nerve of the frog were diminished only slightly by the external application of quaternary ammonium compounds related to lidocaine.[93] However, axoplasmic injection and infusion of these quaternary compounds inhibited sodium currents by more than 90%. On the basis of his studies, Strichartz has suggested that the receptor site for these quaternary ammonium compounds related to lidocaine is located halfway down the electrical gradient from the inside to the outside of the sodium channel. Hille, Courtney, and Dunn have presented evidence based on similar studies that the receptor site for tertiary amine local anesthetic drugs such as lidocaine is the same as that determined for the quaternary ammonium derivatives of these clinically useful local anesthetic agents.[92]

Membrane Reactive Sites

The evidence presented above has been interpreted by most investigators as suggestive of a receptor site for local anesthetic agents. However, alternative theories not involving a specific receptor have been proposed. Zipf has suggested that local anesthetic agents do not necessarily bind with specific receptors on the cell membrane, but rather may interact with ubiquitous-type reactive sites.[95] The inhibition of conduction by local anesthetic agents then could be explained by a surface charge hypothesis.[96] This hypothesis suggests that the interaction of local anesthetic agents with these ubiquitous reactor sites results in the neutralization of the fixed negative charges in the cell membrane such that the potential across the membrane would rise although the recorded resting potential would remain constant. When this increase in the transmembrane potential is sufficiently great, electrotonic currents from neighboring unanesthetized nerve membranes would be insufficient to reduce the membrane potential to its threshold or firing level and conduction blockade would then occur.

Membrane Expansion

Although the cationic form of agents such as lidocaine, mepivacaine, prilocaine, and bupivacaine appears to be responsible for their local anesthetic action, other compounds are known to exist as uncharged molecules at physiological pH and still exert clinically useful anesthetic activity. Benzocaine, for example, does not exist in the cationic form and yet exhibits potent topical anesthetic properties. Studies by Ritchie and Ritchie on the relationship of pH to the conduction blocking properties of benzocaine have revealed that the anesthetic activity of benzocaine is unaffected by changes in pH.[97] It is difficult to conceive that such uncharged molecules could act at a specific receptor site in the same fashion as the cationic form of the conventional local anesthetic agents.

The membrane expansion theory, which actually preceded the specific receptor theory, has been reproposed as a possible explanation for the local anesthetic activity of compounds such as benzocaine. The original form of this theory postulated an increased lateral pressure in the membrane by local anesthetic agents, which could produce a constriction of the membrane channels through which sodium ions move.[70] In vitro studies by Skou, in which the surface pressure of monomolecular layers of lipids increased following placement of local anesthetic drugs into the solution below the lipid layers, served as the basis for this form of the membrane expansion theory.[98-100] More recently, Johnson and Murphy have suggested that an increased movement of lipid molecules produces a confirmational change in proteins associated with lipids in the cell membrane resulting in an expansion of the membrane.[101] Support for this view of the membrane expansion theory was presented by Seeman, who observed an inverse correlation between the membrane-buffer partition coefficient and membrane concentration required for conduction blockade of agents which exist mainly in the uncharged form.[102] These data have been interpreted as indicating that compounds which are highly lipid soluble can penetrate the lipid portion of the cell membrane more readily, causing a confirmational change in the lipoprotein matrix of the membrane, with a resultant decrease in the diameter of the sodium channels, which thereby results in an inhibition of sodium conductance and neural excitation.

Classification of Local Anesthetic Agents by Site of Action

Takman has proposed a biological classification of local anesthetic agents based on information currently available regarding site of action of local anesthetic drugs and the active form of these compounds[103] (Table 7). According to this classification, local anesthetic compounds can be categorized as follows:

Table 7

CLASSIFICATION OF LOCAL ANESTHETIC SUBSTANCES ACCORDING TO BIOLOGICAL SITE AND MODE OF ACTION

Classification	Definition	Chemical Substances
Class A	Agents acting at receptor site on external surface of nerve membrane.	Tetrodotoxin Saxitoxin
Class B	Agents acting at receptor site on internal surface of nerve membrane.	Quaternary ammonium analogues of lidocaine, e.g.
Class C	Agents acting by a receptor independent physicochemical mechanism.	Benzocaine N-butanol Benzylalcohol
Class D	Agents acting by a combination of a receptor and receptor independent mechanism.	Most clinically useful local anesthetic agents, e.g. lidocaine mepivacaine prilocaine

Class A. Agents acting at a receptor site on the *external* surface of the sodium channel: tetrodotoxin, saxitoxin.

Class B. Agents acting at a receptor at the *internal* axoplasmic opening of the sodium channel: quaternary ammonium compounds, e.g., QX 314, QX 572, QX 222.

Class C. Agents acting by way of a receptor independent mechanism: benzocaine, N-butanol, benzylalcohol.

Class D. Agents acting both via a receptor mechanism and a receptor independent mechanism, i.e., procaine, lidocaine, mepivacaine, prilocaine, bupivacaine, and etidocaine.

Class A and B contain compounds that exist only in a charged form such as the biotoxins and quaternary ammonium analogues of lidocaine. The compounds in Class C are chemical substances which exist only in an uncharged form, such as benzocaine. The agents in Class D are anesthetic drugs that can exist in both a charged and uncharged form. Most of the clinically useful local anesthetic agents are in the last category. This classification implies that agents such as lidocaine and mepivacaine would exert their local anesthetic activity both by way of a cationic-receptor site interaction and by a base physicochemical disturbance within the nerve membrane. On the basis of studies carried out on the squid giant axon, Narahashi and Frazier suggested that approximately 90% of the blocking effects of agents such as lidocaine was due to the cationic form of the drug and approximately 10% of the blocking action was caused by the base form.[104]

SUMMARY

1. Peripheral nerves are enclosed in connective tissue sheaths, the endoneurium, perineurium, and epineurium, which act as barriers through which local anesthetic agents must diffuse. In addition, the presence of a myelin sheath in some nerve fibers and a cell membrane, which are basically lipoprotein in nature, also affects the action of anesthetic drugs.
2. Neural excitation is associated with a depolarization and re-polarization of the cell membrane. The depolarization phase re-sults from an increased membrane permeability to sodium ions, whereas the main determinant of the repolarization phase is in-creased potassium conductance.
3. Local anesthetic agents inhibit neural excitation by impeding sodium conductance, which thereby prevents membrane de-polarization.
4. Most of the clinically useful local anesthetic drugs probably act by displacement of calcium from a lipoprotein receptor site lo-

cated on the internal surface of the cell membrane. This anesthetic-receptor interaction results in blockade of the membrane sodium channel which, in turn, decreases sodium permeability and inhibits membrane depolarization.

5. Most of the clinically useful local anesthetic agents exist in both the charged and uncharged (base) form in solution. The uncharged base form diffuses more readily through neural sheaths, while the charged form is mainly responsible for attachment to the membrane receptor and ultimate blockade of neural activity.

6. The relative proportion of charged and uncharged form is dependent upon the pK_a of the chemical substance, pH of the anesthetic solution, and pH at the injection site. These factors will affect the pharmacological profile of different agents such as onset time, anesthetic potency, and duration of action.

3
Preclinical Aspects of Local Anesthesia

IN VITRO STUDIES

The concentration of drug required to inhibit nerve conduction has been used to define the intrinsic anesthetic potency of a chemical substance. In an attempt to compare the relative potency of different anesthetic agents, the concept of minimum anesthetic concentration (Cm) was introduced and defined as the minimum concentration of local anesthetic agent necessary to block impulse conduction in a nerve fiber of given diameter within a reasonable period of time.[1] Cm was intended to be comparable to the minimum alveolar concentration (MAC) of general inhalation anesthetic agents and so could serve as a means of grading relative potency. Unfortunately, differences in experimental techniques and definitions make it impossible to compare the Cm values as reported by various investigators.

Experimental Models

In vitro isolated nerve preparations have been employed by most investigators to determine the conduction blocking activity of specific chemical compounds. Although the electrode configuration used may differ from laboratory to laboratory, the type of apparatus commonly utilized to study nerve conduction consists essentially of a series of electrodes on which an isolated nerve can be placed (Fig. 3-1).[105-107] One segment of the nerve can be stimulated electrically with square wave pulses of varying intensity, duration, and frequency, and surface action potentials can be recorded from the opposite end. A

41

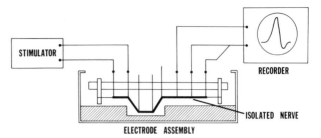

Fig. 3-1.   Diagram of experimental apparatus for isolated nerve studies.

segment of the nerve between the stimulating and recording electrodes is bathed with the local anesthetic solution. The sequential electrical events which occur following exposure of that segment of the nerve to local anesthetic agents consist of (1) a prolongation of the time interval between the stimulus artifact and the action potential, which indicates delayed conduction through the bathed segment and (2) a decrease in the height of the action potential, which indicates complete block of conduction in individual nerve fibers (Fig. 3-2).[108] Most studies have utilized the local anesthetic concentration required to reduce the amplitude of the surface action potential within a specific time period as a measure of intrinsic anesthetic potency. How-

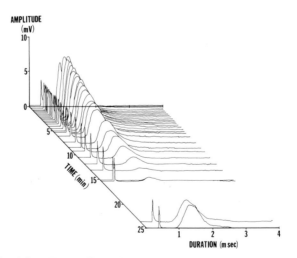

Fig. 3-2.   Three dimensional action potential response of isolated frog sciatic nerve to 5 mM lidocaine.[108] (Courtesy of Dr. Meymaris.)

ever, markedly different potency values have been reported for the same agent depending upon the desired reduction of the amplitude of the action potential and the desired "specific time". For example, the reported concentrations of lidocaine which will produce a significant depression of the action potential amplitude in an isolated nerve preparation vary from 0.25 to 20 mM,[20,41,71,76,97,107,109,110] depending on the end point of amplitude depression, time of exposure to local anesthetic solution, pH of bathing solution, intensity and frequency of nerve stimulation, and type of nerve preparation.

The degree of depression of the action potential amplitude selected to evaluate anesthetic activity can markedly alter the relative Cm values. A 50% suppression in action potential height of the sheathed frog sciatic nerve can be achieved by 5 minutes exposure to 5 mM lidocaine. An 80% depression requires 10 mM and complete suppression is achieved within 5 minutes with 20 mM lidocaine (Fig. 3-3). If the degree of amplitude depression is maintained constant and the time required to produce the desired reduction is altered, then the

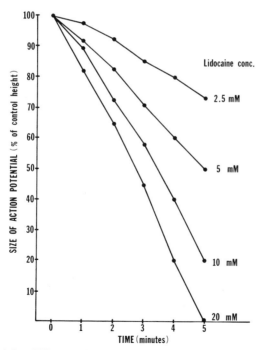

Fig. 3-3. Effect of local anesthetic concentration on rate of conduction blockade.

Cm value again will vary. A 50% suppression in amplitude can be achieved in 5 minutes by the use of a 5 mM concentration of lidocaine. However, only 2.5 mM of this agent are required to produce the same degree of depression in 10 minutes.

The pH of the bathing solution will influence the Cm value of certain local anesthetic agents. [71, 72, 76, 78, 97] A 50% reduction in amplitude of the desheathed rabbit vagus nerve can be achieved within 10 minutes with 10 mM of dibucaine solution at a pH of 7.2. One hundred mM dibucaine is required to produce the same action potential suppression when the pH of the bathing solution is 9.2.[72] This alteration of anesthetic potency by pH is related to the pK_a of the chemical compound and the proportion of drug present in the base and cationic form (Fig. 3-4). As indicated in Chapter 2, the cationic

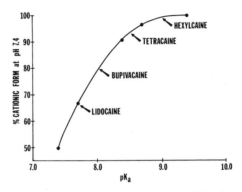

Fig. 3-4.   Relationship of pK_a to percent of local anesthetic agent present in cationic form at pH 7.4.

form of the class D agents, e.g., lidocaine, mepivacaine, is mainly responsible for local anesthetic activity. Therefore, a reduction in pH will produce an increase in the proportion of available cation, which, in turn, will result in an apparent increase in anesthetic potency on desheathed nerves.

The action potential usually recorded from an isolated nerve represents mainly the A spike of the compound action potential. The height of the A spike will vary as a function of the stimulus intensity until a maximum amplitude is achieved indicating all A fibers are firing. The stimulus intensity should be adjusted initially to produce an action potential of maximum height, i.e., the stimulus intensity should be supramaximal. Changes in stimulus intensity must be avoided during the period of exposure to the local anesthetic solution in order to ascertain accurately the conduction blocking effect of the anesthetic agent.

The rate of stimulation will also affect the apparent anesthetic potency (Fig. 3-5). When the stimulus frequency is increased from 3 to 30 pulses/sec, 5 mM lidocaine decreases the amplitude of the A spike to approximately 60% and 50% of its initial height respectively. At a stimulus frequency of 100 pulses/sec, 5 mM of lidocaine will reduce the A spike of the sheathed frog sciatic nerve to approximately 40% of its control height within 5 minutes.

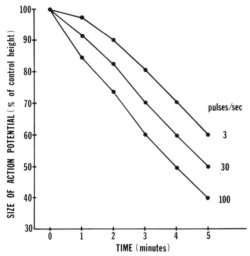

Fig. 3-5. Effect of frequency of stimulation on rate of conduction blockade.

The type of nerve preparation also will influence the observed intrinsic potency. In addition to the frog sciatic nerve, which has been employed most commonly for the in vitro study of anesthetic activity, mammalian nerves such as the rabbit vagus also have been utilized. A comparison of the desheathed frog sciatic nerve and desheathed rabbit vagus nerve reveals a more rapid decrease and a more profound depression of the frog sciatic nerve action potential than of the rabbit vagus following exposure to 300 μM of lidocaine. Moreover, this same concentration of lidocaine was found to exert a much greater depressant effect on the B fibers of the sheathed rabbit vagus nerve as compared to its A fibers.[71] Heavner and de Jong observed that preganglionic B fibers from the rabbit cervical sympathetic trunk, although myelinated, were three times more sensitive to lidocaine than unmyelinated postganglionic C fibers.[111] These findings may have clinical relevance since sympathetic blockade (B fibers) is more extensive than sensory block (C fibers) following spinal anesthesia.

Finally, the presence or absence of the nerve sheath can alter significantly the apparent anesthetic potency of different agents. A desheathed nerve preparation is considerably more sensitive to the conduction blocking action of the commonly used clinical agents such as lidocaine and bupivacaine at a neutral pH.[71, 79] The clinical application of this phenomenon can be appreciated from a comparison of the local anesthetic dosage requirements for spinal and epidural anesthesia. Only 50–100 mg of lidocaine will produce profound anesthesia when administered into the subarachnoid space where the spinal cord is comparable to a desheathed nerve preparation. In the epidural space, where sheathed nerve fibers are present, 200–300 mg of lidocaine are required to attain sensory analgesia similar in quality to spinal anesthesia.

Intrinsic Potency

The commonly used local analgesic agents have been evaluated by determining the minimum concentration (Cm) required to produce a 50–60% reduction in A spike amplitude of the sheathed frog sciatic nerve within 5 minutes in a solution of pH 7.2–7.4 and at a stimulus frequency of 30 pulses/sec. Under these standardized conditions, procaine is the least potent of the agents currently used in clinical practice (Table 8). Chloroprocaine, lidocaine, mepivacaine, and

Table 8

RELATIVE IN VITRO CONDUCTION BLOCKING AND PHYSICAL-CHEMICAL PROPERTIES OF VARIOUS AGENTS

AGENT	RELATIVE CONDUCTION BLOCKING PROPERTIES*			PHYSICAL-CHEMICAL PROPERTIES		
	POTENCY	ONSET	DURATION	pK$_a$	LIPID SOLUBILITY	PROTEIN BINDING
Low Potency						
PROCAINE	1	1	1	8.9	0.6	5.8
Intermediate Potency						
MEPIVACAINE	2	1	1.5	7.6	1.0	77
PRILOCAINE	3	1	1.5	7.7	0.8	55
CHLOROPROCAINE	4	0.8	0.75	8.7	—	—
LIDOCAINE	4	0.8	1.5	7.7	2.9	64
High Potency						
TETRACAINE	16	2	8	8.5	80	76
BUPIVACAINE	16	0.6	8	8.1	28	95
ETIDOCAINE	16	0.4	8	7.7	141	94

*Data derived from isolated frog sciatic nerve

prilocaine may be classified as compounds of intermediate potency, i.e., 2–4 times as potent as procaine. Tetracaine, bupivacaine, and etidocaine represent drugs of high potency which are approximately 20 times more active than procaine. Tetrodotoxin is the most potent conduction blocking substance studied to date. Eighty nmoles of this compound will produce a 50% reduction in the amplitude of the surface action potential of the desheathed rabbit vagus nerve.[112, 113] This would indicate that tetrodotoxin has an intrinsic anesthetic potency which is approximately 250,000 times greater than that of procaine.

Onset of Conduction Blockade

One of the important clinical parameters in regional anesthesia is the rapidity with which conduction blockade occurs. This pharmacological property of local anesthetic agents can be evaluated quite accurately in an isolated nerve preparation. The relative latency of the clinically useful analgesic agents has been determined in a standardized manner, i.e., the concentration required to produce a 50% reduction in the height of the sheathed frog sciatic nerve action potential within 10 minutes. A correlation was believed to exist between the potency, duration, and onset time of local anesthetic agents. Agents of high potency and long duration of action such as tetracaine and dibucaine have historically shown the slowest onset of anesthesia.[20] However, the introduction of newer agents of high potency and long duration of action such as bupivacaine and etidocaine indicates that no correlation exists between the onset of action of various chemical compounds and their intrinsic anesthetic potency or duration of activity.[43] In fact, etidocaine possesses the most rapid onset time and tetracaine shows the longest latency (Table 8). Onset time is probably related to the physicochemical properties of these various agents, e.g., pK_a and lipid solubility. For example, a comparison of agents with similar pK_a values such as lidocaine, prilocaine, and etidocaine reveals that the most lipid-soluble drug, etidocaine, demonstrates the most rapid onset of action whereas the least lipid-soluble agent, prilocaine, has the longest latency. Lidocaine occupies an intermediate position both in terms of lipid solubility and onset time. A comparison of highly lipid-soluble compounds with varying pK_a values, e.g., etidocaine, bupivacaine, and tetracaine, indicates that etidocaine, which possesses the lowest pK_a, has the most rapid onset of action, whereas tetracaine possesses the highest pK_a value and the slowest onset time. The pK_a and latency values for bupivacaine lie between the two extremes. [20, 114, 115] These observations concerning onset time are consistent with the known relationships between pH, pK_a, relative proportion of analgesic agents in the base and cationic form, lipid solubility, and lipid composition of the cell membrane.

Duration of Action

In an isolated nerve preparation, conduction blockade will persist as long as the nerve remains exposed to the local anesthetic containing solution. Duration of action in vitro usually is determined in the following manner: following exposure of an isolated nerve for a period sufficient to reduce the surface action potential by 50%, the local anesthetic solution is removed. The nerve then is bathed with a normal Ringer's solution. The time required for the action potential to return to its control amplitude is a measure of the duration of action of the local anesthetic agent. It is necessary to use equipotent concentrations of local anesthetic drugs when comparing their relative durations of action, since the duration of conduction blockade with any single agent varies as a function of the anesthetic concentration of that agent. [116] The clinically useful analgesic drugs can be classified essentially into two categories based on their in vitro durations of action: agents of short duration, i.e., 15 to 30 minutes are required for complete recovery, and agents of long duration, i.e., 100 to 150 minutes are required for complete recovery. Procaine, chloroprocaine, lidocaine, mepivacaine, and prilocaine fall into the first category whereas tetracaine, bupivacaine, and etidocaine are agents possessing a long duration of action. In general, those compounds belonging to the short-duration class possess relatively low lipid solubility and low protein-binding characteristics. Agents of long duration are characterized by high lipid solubility and high protein-binding properties (Table 8).

IN VIVO ANIMAL STUDIES

Models

A number of animal models have been utilized to evaluate the pharmacological profile of local anesthetic agents in vivo. [107] Intradermal wheals have been performed mainly in guinea pigs as an example of infiltration anesthesia. [12, 88, 116-119] Sciatic nerve blocks in rats and brachial plexus blocks in guinea pigs have been employed for peripheral nerve blockade.[12, 88, 90, 106, 110, 119] In recent years, techniques for producing epidural anesthesia in guinea pigs, cats, dogs, and sheep have been developed.[90, 120, 121] In addition, spinal anesthesia in rabbits, dogs, and sheep has been utilized as a model for central neural blockade.[110, 122-124] Local anesthetic solutions have been applied to the rabbit cornea and instilled intratracheally in rabbits to evaluate the topical anesthetic activity of various compounds.[106, 110, 119] With these various techniques, it is possible to determine frequency of anesthesia, onset time, and duration of action.

Anesthetic Potency

The in vivo anesthetic potency of local anesthetic agents may differ from their intrinsic potency as determined by in vitro techniques. This may be due to other factors such as vasodilation and/or physiological disposition. For example, the intrinsic potency of chloroprocaine is approximately 4 times greater than that of procaine in an in vitro system (Table 9). However, in vivo studies

Table 9

COMPARATIVE INTRINSIC ANESTHETIC POTENCY AND IN VIVO Cm OF VARIOUS
LOCAL ANESTHETIC AGENTS

AGENT	RELATIVE INTRINSIC POTENCY	Cm * RAT SCIATIC NERVE	Cm ** CAT EPIDURAL ANESTHESIA
PROCAINE	1	1.0	4.0
MEPIVACAINE	2	0.5	2.0
PRILOCAINE	3	0.5	2.0
CHLOROPROCAINE	4	1.0	2.0
LIDOCAINE	4	0.5	2.0
BUPIVACAINE	16	0.125	0.5
ETIDOCAINE	16	0.125	0.5
TETRACAINE	16	0.125	0.5

*Cm = minimum concentration (0.2ml) required to produce 50% anesthetic frequency.
**Cm = minimum concentration (1.5ml) required to produce 50% frequency of flexor reflex blockade.

suggest that the equieffective concentration of these two agents is the same. This finding may be related to the extremely rapid hydrolysis of chloroprocaine as compared to procaine. Similarly, the intrinsic potency of lidocaine has been shown to be approximately 1.5–2 times greater than that of mepivacaine and prilocaine (Table 9), whereas animal data indicate that the concentrations of these three agents required to produce equivalent anesthetic activity are similar when used for sciatic nerve blocks in rats or spinal anesthesia in rabbits.[88, 110] This apparent discrepancy between in vivo and in vitro anesthetic potency may be attributable to a greater vasodilator action of lidocaine, which results in a more rapid vascular absorption and decreased availability of this agent for neural uptake. With regard to compounds in the high potency group, bupivacaine and etidocaine possess the same Cm in terms of conduction blockade in the isolated frog sciatic nerve preparation.[114, 115] However, epidural studies in sheep indicate that 1% etidocaine is required to produce anesthetic results comparable to those achieved with 0.75% bupivacaine.[121] This difference may be due to the greater lipid solubility of etidocaine, which causes this agent to be sequestered in peridural fat with fewer molecules available for neural uptake. A comparison of the relative in vitro and in vivo anesthetic potency of the various clinically useful agents is presented in Table 9.

Topical anesthetic potency may differ from the in vivo anesthetic potency which is obtained following injection of agents in the region of nerve endings or fibers. Block of the corneal reflex in rabbits and guinea pigs has been used most frequently to evaluate the topical anesthetic properties of different agents.[107] Other techniques such as blockade of the sneeze reflex in rabbits have also been employed.[110] A comparison of the topical anesthetic potency of various local anesthetic compounds as evaluated in animal preparations indicates that tetracaine and cocaine demonstrate the most potent topical anesthetic activity, followed in order of decreasing potency by etidocaine, bupivacaine, lidocaine, and prilocaine. Interestingly, procaine and mepivacaine, which possess easily measureable anesthetic activity when administered by injection, provide only minimal surface anesthesia when applied topically. The precise reason for the poor topical anesthetic properties of these two agents has not been completely elucidated.

Onset and Duration of Action

It is difficult to differentiate between the onset time of various agents in animal models. Usually, onset of anesthesia occurs quite rapidly when the various compounds are employed in equieffective concentrations. Differences in onset time can be determined when epidural anesthesia is performed in animals such as cats, dogs, or sheep. Duce and co-workers demonstrated in cats that the onset of epidural anesthesia with lidocaine is decreased with an increased dose.[120] Addition of epinephrine and alteration in the pH of the local anesthetic solution produced inconsistent changes in latency. Equieffective concentrations of lidocaine and tetracaine showed similar onset times.

The duration of motor block can be determined quite accurately in animals. On the basis of various types of peripheral or central neural blocks in different animal species, local anesthetic agents can be categorized as compounds of short, moderate, long, or ultralong duration of action. Procaine and chloroprocaine represent drugs of short duration of action both for peripheral nerve blockade and central neural blockade in animals. Lidocaine, mepivacaine, and prilocaine possess a moderate duration of action while tetracaine, bupivacaine, and etidocaine can be classified as agents of long duration of action. Tetrodotoxin and saxitoxin demonstrate ultralong anesthetic activity (Table 10).

Table 10

DURATION OF SPINAL ANESTHESIA IN SHEEP OF LIDOCAINE (50mg), TETRACAINE (10mg) AND TETRODOTOXIN (4 μg).

	LIDOCAINE	TETRACAINE	TETRODOTOXIN
DIGITAL PAIN	36 - 42 min	60 - 140 min	17 - 23 hrs
WEIGHT SUPPORT	38 - 60 min	165 - 202 min	17 - 23 hrs
FULL RECOVERY	60 - 85 min	282 - 405 min	25 - 28 hrs
n = 4			

The duration of local analgesia can be altered by factors such as the dosage of the agent and the addition of a vasoconstrictor substance, e.g., epinephrine, to the local anesthetic solution. Figure 3-6 depicts the dose-duration response curve for several agents employed for rat sciatic nerve blocks and epidural anesthesia in cats. [12, 120] An increase in duration of action occurs as the dosage is increased until a maximum value is reached or systemic toxicity occurs. The prolongation of analgesic activity bears a closer relationship to the total dosage than to concentration or volume of solution employed (Table 11).

Depending on the site of administration, vasoconstrictor agents can markedly increase the frequency of successful nerve blocks and prolong the duration of action of local anesthetic agents (Table 12). [88, 120, 125] The mechanism of this increased frequency and duration of anesthesia is related to a localized vasoconstriction in the area of administration, which results in a decreased systemic absorption of

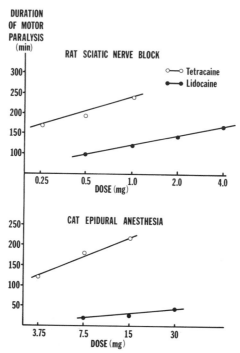

Fig. 3-6. Dose-duration relationship of tetracaine and lidocaine following rat sciatic nerve block and cat epidural anesthesia.

Table 11

ONSET AND DURATION OF HIND LIMB PARALYSIS IN CATS FOLLOWING EPIDURAL ADMINISTRATION OF VARYING VOLUMES, CONCENTRATIONS AND DOSAGE OF LIDOCAINE SOLUTIONS.

DOSE (mg)	15	15	30	30
CONCENTRATION (%)	1.0	1.5	1.5	2.0
VOLUME (ml)	1.5	1.0	2.0	1.5
ONSET (min) Mean ± S.D.	4.1 ± 0.9	5.9 ± 0.9	3.0 ± 0.9	2.4 ± 0.5
DURATION (min) Mean ± S.D.	22.1 ± 3.7	22.7 ± 5.7	35.7 ± 7.3	43.6 ± 5.6

Table 12

EFFECT OF EPINEPHRINE ON THE FREQUENCY AND DURATION OF PERIPHERAL AND CENTRAL NEURAL BLOCKADE

AGENT	ANESTHETIC PROCEDURE	WITHOUT EPINEPHRINE		WITH EPINEPHRINE	
		FREQUENCY OF COMPLETE BLOCK	DURATION OF ANESTHESIA (min)	FREQUENCY OF COMPLETE BLOCK	DURATION OF ANESTHESIA (min)
0.5% LIDOCAINE	CAT EPIDURAL ANESTHESIA	31.8%	20.4 ± 1.0	100%	32 ± 7.8
0.125% LIDOCAINE + TETRODOTOXIN 2 µg/ml	RAT SCIATIC NERVE BLOCK	20%	174	100%	368 ± 24

the anesthetic compound such that more of the agent is available for diffusion into neural tissue. Epinephrine is the agent usually added to local anesthetic solutions for the purpose of providing a localized state of vasoconstriction. Other sympathomimetic vasoconstrictor agents such as norepinephrine and phenylephrine also have been utilized to improve the frequency and duration of regional anesthesia (Table 13).[125] Nonsympathomimetic amine agents such as octapressin have also been studied as vasoconstrictor supplements for local anesthetic agents. Animal studies by Åkerman indicate that 0.9 µg/ml of octapressin may be equivalent to 3.33–5.0 µg/ml of epinephrine in terms of its ability to retard the absorption and prolong the anesthetic activity of lidocaine and prilocaine.[126]

Onset and duration of action can be altered by combining agents of rapid onset and short or moderate duration with substances possessing slow onset, but long or ultralong activity. Combinations of procaine or lidocaine with tetracaine or tetrodotoxin have been studied in animals, and the results suggest that the anesthetic mixture

Table 13

EFFECT OF VARIOUS VASOCONSTRICTOR AGENTS ON THE DURATION OF RAT SCIATIC NERVE BLOCKS PRODUCED BY 0.125% LIDOCAINE + 2µg/ml TETRODOTOXIN.

VASOCONSTRICTOR AGENT	CONCENTRATION	FREQUENCY OF COMPLETE BLOCK	DURATION (min)
NONE	—	20%	174
EPINEPHRINE	1 : 200,000	100%	368 ± 24
NOREPINEPHRINE	1 : 20,000	100%	354 ± 12
PHENYLEPHRINE	1 : 20,000	100%	377 ± 27

Table 14

EFFECT OF LOCAL ANESTHETIC MIXTURES ON ONSET TIME AND
DURATION OF EPIDURAL ANESTHESIA IN DOGS

AGENTS	ONSET TIME (min)	DURATION (min)
1.0% LIDOCAINE	2.02 ± 0.33	123.8 ± 6.8
0.2% TETRACAINE	4.0 ± 0.66	272.4 ± 27.4
1.0% LIDOCAINE + 0.2% TETRACAINE	2.0 ± 0.20	282.7 ± 23.1

will possess the most favorable properties of the individual agents, i.e., rapid onset and long duration (Table 14).[125, 127] More detailed information concerning the relative onset and duration of local analgesic agents and the various factors which may influence their pharmacological properties can be obtained from studies in man (Chapter 4).

SUMMARY

1. The intrinsic anesthetic potency of a chemical compound is usually defined as the minimum concentration required to produce within 5–10 minutes a 50% reduction in the amplitude of the surface action potential recorded from an isolated nerve preparation.
2. Intrinsic anesthetic potency (Cm) may be influenced in vitro by various factors such as frequency and intensity of stimulation, type of isolated nerve preparation, presence or absence of a neural sheath and pH of anesthetic solution.
3. The clinically useful agents can be categorized as compounds of (a) low potency, e.g., procaine; (b) moderate potency, e.g., mepivacaine, prilocaine, chloroprocaine, and lidocaine; and (c) high potency, e.g., tetracaine, bupivacaine, and etidocaine.
4. Onset and duration of conduction blockade are related to pK_a, lipid solubility, and protein binding. In general, a lower pK_a and higher lipid solubility are associated with a more rapid onset time, while a higher protein-binding capacity is related to a longer duration of action.
5. The relative in vivo anesthetic potency, onset, and duration of different agents are similar to, but not identical with, in vitro

results. The observed differences betweeen in vitro and in vivo properties are due to other pharmacological actions of local analgesic drugs, such as vasodilation.

6. On the basis of in vivo animal studies, the various agents may be classified according to their relative durations of action, i.e., (a) short duration, e.g., procaine and chloroprocaine; (b) moderate duration, e.g., lidocaine, prilocaine, and mepivacaine; (c) long duration, e.g., tetracaine, bupivacaine, and etidocaine; and (d) ultralong duration, e.g., tetrodotoxin and saxitoxin.

4

Clinical Aspects of
Local Anesthesia

GENERAL COMMENTS

Local anesthetic requirements and activity vary considerably, depending on such factors as anesthetic procedure, surgical procedure, and physiological status of the patient.[128] It is unlikely that any single chemical compound can provide sufficient versatility for all clinical conditions. Thus, selection of an appropriate agent in a specific situation requires knowledge of the clinical needs and the pharmacological properties of the various anesthetic drugs currently available. The regional anesthetic procedure itself probably exerts the greatest influence on the type of agent to be used, due mainly to the marked anatomical and physiological differences between various sites of administration. Primarily on the basis of anatomical considerations, regional anesthesia may be divided into four categories: infiltration, peripheral nerve blockade, central neural blockade, and topical anesthesia (Table 15). Infiltration anesthesia involves inhibition of excitation primarily at nerve endings. Peripheral nerve blockade impedes conduction in nerve fibers of the peripheral nervous system. Central neural blockade interferes with conduction in nerve fibers considered to be part of the central nervous system. Topical anesthesia requires diffusion through tissue barriers such as skin or mucous membranes to peripheral nerve endings where inhibition of excitation occurs.

Variations in anesthetic activity may occur as a function of many conditions, e.g., (1) the regional procedure employed, (2) the physical or clinical status of the patient, (3) factors associated with the surgical procedure or (4) the composition of the anesthetic solution.

Table 15

CLASSIFICATION OF REGIONAL ANESTHESIA

1. INFILTRATION
   a. EXTRAVASCULAR
   b. INTRAVASCULAR

2. PERIPHERAL NERVE BLOCKADE
   a. MINOR NERVE BLOCKADE, i.e. SINGLE NERVE BLOCK
   b. MAJOR NERVE BLOCKADE, i.e. MULTIPLE NERVE BLOCK
      OR PLEXUS BLOCKADE

3. CENTRAL NEURAL BLOCKADE
   a. EPIDURAL BLOCKADE
      1. THORACIC
      2. LUMBAR
      3. CAUDAL
   b. SUBARACHNOID BLOCK

4. TOPICAL ANESTHESIA

Differences in anesthetic activity as a function of the regional procedure are demonstrated in Table 16 in which the properties of lidocaine and bupivacaine are compared.[129-134] Onset of action occurs immediately in infiltration anesthesia, whereas the longest latency (14–23 minutes) is observed in peripheral nerve blockade of the multiple nerve type, e.g., brachial plexus block. The shortest duration of anesthesia for most agents occurs in central neural blocks of the subarachnoid type. The duration of action at other sites, however, depends upon the local anesthetic agent used. For example, duration of action persists for the longest period following percutaneous infiltration for an agent such as lidocaine, whereas the longest duration of bupivacaine is observed when it is administered for peripheral nerve

Table 16

ONSET AND DURATION OF ACTION OF LIDOCAINE AND BUPIVACAINE
FOLLOWING VARIOUS FORMS OF REGIONAL ANESTHESIA

ANESTHETIC PROCEDURE	LIDOCAINE			BUPIVACAINE		
	SOLUTION	SENSORY ONSET (min)	SENSORY DURATION (min)	SOLUTION	SENSORY ONSET (min)	SENSORY DURATION (min)
1. INFILTRATION a. EXTRAVASCULAR	1% w/epi 1:200,000	—	416.2 ± 25.8	0.25% w/epi 1:200,000	—	428.6 ± 39.9
b. INTRAVENOUS REGIONAL	0.5%	—	111.0 ± 26.6	0.25%	—	344.0 ± 27.7
2. PERIPHERAL NERVE BLOCKADE a. ULNAR NERVE BLOCK	1% w/epi 1:200,000	3.00±0.5	178.0 ± 17	0.25% w/epi 1:200,000	16.00 ± 4.7	395.0 ± 22
b. BRACHIAL PLEXUS BLOCK	1% w/epi 1:200,000	14.04±3.83	195.0 ± 26.3	0.25% w/epi 1:200,000	23.26 ± 7.93	613.0 ±126
3. CENTRAL NEURAL BLOCKADE a. EPIDURAL	2% w/epi 1:200,000	5.07±0.58	156.6 ± 15	0.5 % w/epi 1:200,000	6.27 ± 1.19	228.6 ± 23
b. SUBARACHNOID	5%	4.30±1.5	94.0 ± 28	1%	30 - 90 sec	128.0 ± 19

block, e.g., brachial plexus blockade. Bupivacaine demonstrates a fivefold difference in anesthetic duration depending on the type of regional anesthetic procedure, e.g., 128 minutes of spinal anesthesia as compared to 613 minutes of brachial plexus blockade.[131-134]

The physical and clinical status of a patient can markedly affect local anesthetic activity. The dose requirements of local anesthetic agents may be altered by patient characteristics, e.g., the dose per segment requirement of local analgesic drugs administered epidurally has been reported to be inversely proportional to age, stage of pregnancy, and degree of arteriosclerosis and directly proportional to the height of the patient (Table 17).[135] Duration of infiltration anesthesia and peripheral nerve blockade also may be influenced by the clinical status of the patient. The expected duration of lidocaine for brachial plexus blockade was significantly shorter in subjects with chronic renal failure,[136] whereas the duration of infiltration anesthesia and digital nerve block with lidocaine was prolonged markedly in patients with scleroderma.[137, 138] In general, the activity of amide-type agents may be prolonged in the presence of severe liver dysfunction and the action of ester-type drugs may be enhanced if a deficiency of the enzyme, pseudocholinesterase, exists. In either situation, a decreased rate of degradation and elimination of the local anesthetic agent would occur.

Factors associated with the surgical procedure also may affect local anesthetic activity. A significantly longer duration of pain relief has been observed in patients treated with lidocaine when two or more units of blood were lost during surgery.[139] Blood loss may result in hypotension and a reflex state of generalized vasoconstriction, which decreases the absorption of local anesthetic agents from their injection site and prolongs the duration of anesthesia.

Table 17

INFLUENCE OF PATIENT STATUS ON LOCAL ANESTHETIC ACTIVITY

PATIENT STATUS	INFILTRATION ANESTHESIA	PERIPHERAL NERVE BLOCKADE	EPIDURAL ANESTHESIA
PREGNANCY	—	—	↑ ANESTHETIC SPREAD
ARTERIOSCLEROSIS	—	—	↑ ANESTHETIC SPREAD
RENAL FAILURE	—	↓ DURATION	—
SCLERODERMA	↑ DURATION	↑ DURATION	—
LIVER DISEASE	↑ DURATION OF AMIDE-TYPE AGENTS	↑ DURATION OF AMIDE-TYPE AGENTS	↑ DURATION OF AMIDE-TYPE AGENTS
PSEUDOCHOLINESTERASE DEFICIENCY	↑ DURATION OF ESTER AGENTS	↑ DURATION OF ESTER AGENTS	↑ DURATION OF ESTER AGENTS

Table 18

EFFECT OF SOLUTION COMPOSITION ON ANESTHETIC ACTIVITY

	ONSET OF ANESTHESIA	DURATION OF ANESTHESIA	FREQUENCY OF ANESTHESIA
↑DOSAGE (vol. or conc.)	↓	↑	↑
VASOCONSTRICTOR AGENT	↓—	↑	↑
METHYLPARABEN	—	—	—
SODIUM METABISULFITE	—	—	—
CO_2	↓	—	—
EXCESS K^+	↓	↑	—

The composition of the solution employed can influence the primary pharmacological activity of the anesthetic agent (Table 18). An increase in anesthetic dosage will decrease the onset time and increase both duration and frequency of satisfactory analgesia[140] (Fig. 4-1). This dose-related effect may be achieved by alterations in either

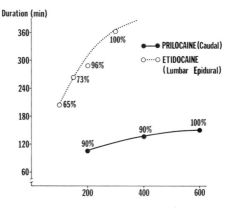

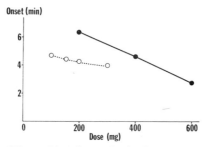

Fig. 4-1. Effect of local anesthetic dosage on onset, duration, and frequency of analgesia.

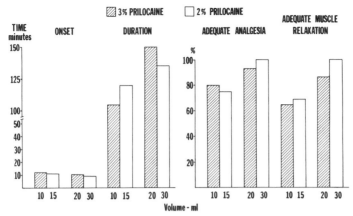

Fig. 4-2.   Influence of concentration and volume of anesthetic solution on various anesthetic parameters.

volume or concentration[141] (Fig. 4-2). Vasoconstrictor agents, usually epinephrine, frequently are added to local anesthetic solutions to decrease the rate of drug absorption from the site of injection and prolong the duration of anesthesia. Such prolongation of anesthesia by epinephrine is dependent on the local analgesic agent and the type

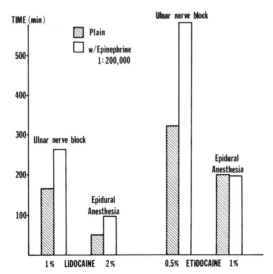

Fig. 4-3.   Influence of epinephrine on the anesthetic duration of lidocaine and etidocaine in ulnar nerve blockade and epidural anesthesia.

of regional procedure. Epinephrine will extend significantly the action of agents such as procaine and lidocaine for infiltration, peripheral, and central neural blockade.[129, 135, 142, 143] A prolongation of local anesthetic activity may occur when prilocaine, bupivacaine, and etidocaine are combined with epinephrine for peripheral nerve blockade,[142] whereas the duration of epidural anesthesia with these agents is not altered by the addition of a vasoconstrictor drug[135, 143–145] (Fig. 4-3).

Local anesthetic solutions may contain other ingredients such as methylparaben, which serves as an antibacterial preservative in multiple dose vials, and sodium metabisulfite, which is employed as an antioxidant in epinephrine-containing solutions. The amount of these substances commonly found in commercial local anesthetic solutions does not exert any influence on the basic analgesic properties of the drug.

INFILTRATION ANESTHESIA

This anesthetic procedure involves administration of a local anesthetic agent into an extravascular or intravascular site and subsequent diffusion to nerve endings where excitation is inhibited.[146] The extravascular form also has been termed percutaneous infiltration. The intravascular form consists of the injection of anesthetic drug into the vasculature of a tourniquet-occluded limb such that the drug cannot enter the central circulatory compartment, but instead diffuses from the peripheral vascular bed to nonvascular tissue such as nerve endings.

Extravascular Infiltration

Intradermal wheals have been utilized to evaluate the infiltrative anesthetic properties of various agents.[129, 147, 148] The infiltration anesthetic potency of the clinically useful drugs is similar to their relative intrinsic anesthetic potencies, i.e., 2% procaine, 1% lidocaine, mepivacaine, and prilocaine, and 0.25% bupivacaine are equivalent in terms of frequency of adequate analgesia. Onset of action is almost immediate for all agents following intradermal or subcutaneous administration. However, the various agents can be differentiated according to duration of infiltration anesthesia (Table 19). Procaine has a short duration, whereas lidocaine, mepivacaine, and prilocaine are agents of moderate duration and bupivacaine

Table 19

COMPARATIVE DURATION OF INFILTRATION ANESTHESIA OF VARIOUS
AGENTS FOLLOWING INTRADERMAL ADMINISTRATION

AGENT	CONC. (%)	DURATION (min ± S.E. or range)	
		Plain	Epinephrine 1:200,000
PROCAINE	0.5	20 (15-30)	56 (15-120)
LIDOCAINE	0.5	75 (30-340)	228 (60-435)
LIDOCAINE	1.0	127.6 ± 17.4	416.2 ± 25.8
MEPIVACAINE	0.5	108 (15-240)	240 (135-315)
PRILOCAINE	1.0	99.1 ± 19.1	288.7 ± 10.2
BUPIVACAINE	0.25	199.5 ± 33.4	428.6 ± 39.9

demonstrates long anesthetic activity. Epinephrine will markedly prolong the duration of infiltration anesthesia of all local anesthetic
agents. However, the duration of anesthesia appears to be prolonged
most dramatically when epinephrine is added to solutions of
lidocaine. For example, plain bupivacaine produces a duration of
analgesia 65% longer than that of plain lidocaine. Addition of epinephrine 1:200,000 significantly extends the duration of both agents, but
no difference in analgesic duration exists between lidocaine and
bupivacaine solutions that contain epinephrine.

The most extensive studies of infiltration anesthesia have been
conducted in the dental field, since infiltration of the gingival mucosa
is frequently performed for many routine dental procedures. Agents
commonly used in dentistry are shown in Table 20.[149, 150] In an
attempt to objectively evaluate the factors that influence pulpal anesthesia, a technique of electrical stimulation of teeth has been

Table 20

LOCAL ANESTHETIC AGENTS COMMONLY EMPLOYED FOR INFILTRATION ANESTHESIA IN DENTISTRY

AGENT	CONC. (%)	EPINEPHRINE CONC.	FREQUENCY OF SATISFACTORY ANALGESIA (%)	DURATION OF SOFT TISSUE ANALGESIA (min ± S.E.)
LIDOCAINE	2	1:100,000	93.9	147±7.4
MEPIVACAINE	2	1:20,000 (Neo-cobefrin)	92.0	140±8.0
MEPIVACAINE	3	NONE	90.2	134.5±16.3
PRILOCAINE	4	NONE	93.0	62± 7.0
PRILOCAINE	4	1:200,000	92.6	124.7± 4.8

employed to determine pain threshold and its modification by local anesthetic agents.[151, 152] There are distinct differences in anesthetic potency between various agents. For example, 3% procaine is required to provide an analgesic frequency comparable to that achieved with 1% lidocaine. When the various agents are employed in equipotent concentrations, the concomitant use of a vasoconstrictor agent (epinephrine) exerts the greatest influence on infiltration anesthetic properties.[151] Although plain procaine was ineffective at a concentration of 2%, the addition of epinephrine (25 μg/ml) resulted in an 80% frequency of satisfactory pulpal anesthesia. The addition of epinephrine to solutions of lidocaine was more efficacious than an increase in the concentration of the anesthetic solution (Fig. 4-4). Use of a 4% concentration of plain lidocaine produced approximately an 80% frequency of satisfactory analgesia. On the other hand, 1% lidocaine which was ineffective as a plain solution provided 100% analgesic frequency when used in combination with 25 μg/ml of epinephrine. In general, epinephrine tends to increase the frequency and duration and shorten the onset time for satisfactory analgesia.

Cowan has compared most of the local anesthetic agents commonly used for infiltration anesthesia in dentistry by means of a standardized minimum dosage technique.[153] Two percent procaine with epinephrine (25 μg/ml, 1:40,000) showed the lowest incidence of satisfactory analgesia (70%). All of the other agents, i.e., lidocaine, mepivacaine, and prilocaine produce satisfactory analgesia for dentistry in 90% to 100% of the cases when administered with a vaso-

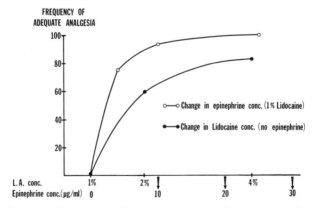

Fig. 4-4. Relative influence of anesthetic concentration and epinephrine on frequency of adequate infiltration anesthesia.

constrictor drug. The importance of a vasoconstrictor agent is also demonstrated by the decrease in frequency of satisfactory analgesia from 90 to 95% to 82% when solutions of 2% mepivacaine with and without epinephrine were compared. As in intradermal wheals, the duration of lidocaine following gingival infiltration is prolonged to a greater extent by the addition of epinephrine than is either mepivacaine or prilocaine. The longest duration of gingival anesthesia was produced by a 2% lidocaine solution containing epinephrine 1:80,000.[153]

Intravascular Infiltration

This form of infiltration anesthesia is commonly referred to as intravenous regional anesthesia or the Bier block in honor of August Bier who initially described this technique in 1908.[154, 155] Numerous articles and several reviews and symposia have been devoted to this topic.[156, 157] The essential features of this procedure are its simplicity and relatively rapid disappearance of analgesia following tourniquet release. The procedure involves the intravascular administration of a local anesthetic agent into a tourniquet-occluded limb. It is imperative that the venous flow from the involved limb be completely obstructed in order to prevent the rapid entrance of local anesthetic drug into the central vascular compartment, which could result in serious toxicity. The type of equipment and the methodology necessary for the safe use of this technique are described in many articles and the requisite precautions should be observed prior to attempting this procedure.

The technique as reported by Bier consisted of exsanguination of the involved extremity by an Esmarch bandage, placement of two elastic bandages, one proximal and one distal to the operative site, and administration of 0.5% procaine into a vein between the two elastic bandages. The method was repopularized in 1963 by Holmes utilizing 0.5% lidocaine as the anesthetic drug.[158]

TECHNICAL CONSIDERATIONS

Although intravenous regional anesthesia is a relatively simple technique, there are a number of factors that may influence both the safety and effectiveness of this procedure.

Tourniquet. Both the safety and efficacy of this regional anesthetic procedure depends on the interruption of blood flow to the involved limb. Calibration of the occlusive cuff is of vital importance since a malfunctioning cuff can lead to inadequate occlusion and potential side effects due to the rapid introduction of local anesthetic agents into the central circulatory compartment.[159] Diffusion of the local anesthetic agent from the intravascular injection site to nonvascular tissue compartments apparently occurs extremely rapidly, since no difference in venous blood levels of the local anesthetic agent could be observed in the occluded limb, following tourniquet release, when the total time of circulatory occlusion was varied between 5 and 100 minutes.[160, 161] A technique of intermittent tourniquet release has been advocated as a means of increasing the safety of this procedure, although there is considerable difference of opinion on the value of this form of tourniquet release. Since peak blood levels of local anesthetic agents occur within 30 sec following cuff deflation, the cyclic deflation/inflation procedure should take place at 10–15 sec intervals in order to decrease the peak levels of local anesthetic drug in the central circulatory compartment. Use of a double pneumatic cuff has also been advocated as an additional safety precaution and as a means of decreasing ischemic pain associated with the tourniquet.

Preinjection Exsanguination. Exsanguination of the involved limb appears to be of value from a safety and efficacy point of view since less drug is required to achieve adequate anesthesia if the limb has been exsanguinated prior to injection. Most commonly, the extremity is elevated to ensure gravity drainage and then tightly wrapped in an Esmarch bandage.

Preinjection Ischemia. Bell, Slater, and Harris have advocated the use of a 20-minute period of ischemia between the time of tourniquet inflation and injection of the local anesthetic solution.[162] This period of preinjection ischemia significantly decreased the dosage of lidocaine required to produce satisfactory surgical analgesia from 3.0 mg/kg to 1.5 mg/kg. Therefore, preinjection ischemia has been advocated as a means of increasing the safety of IV regional anesthesia without sacrificing the quality of analgesia. An increase in tissue pCO_2 and decrease in tissue pH are probably responsible for the increased effectiveness of low doses of local anesthetic agents employed when an adequate period of preinjection ischemia is utilized. The disadvantage of this specific procedure is the increase in patient discomfort during the period of ischemia.[163]

Injection Site. The majority of studies of intravenous regional anesthesia have involved surgical procedures on the upper limbs.[156, 157, 163] It is considerably more difficult to obtain a satisfactory degree of surgical analgesia with this technique in the lower limbs due to the greater mass of tissue involved. In addition, considerably more drug may be required for lower limb procedures, which is a consideration in terms of the safety aspects of this technique.[164] The particular blood vessel in the occluded area chosen for injection does not appear to influence the adequacy of analgesia.[165]

DRUG-RELATED CONSIDERATIONS

Any of the clinically available local anesthetic agents may be utilized for intravascular infiltration anesthesia (Table 21).[163, 166-168] Approximately 18,000 cases of IV regional anesthesia have been reported in the published literature. Lidocaine was the agent utilized in approximately 15,000 patients described in these various studies. Prilocaine, mepivacaine, chloroprocaine, procaine, bupivacaine, and etidocaine also have been used successfully for the production of intravascular regional anesthesia. However, thrombophlebitis has been reported in several patients in whom chloroprocaine was utilized. This phenomenon was not observed with lidocaine or prilocaine in the same study.[166] A relationship does exist between the basic anesthetic properties of the various agents and the duration of analgesia persisting after tourniquet release (Table 21). Residual analgesia following cuff deflation persists for approximately 1–2 hours with agents such as prilocaine and lidocaine, whereas durations of residual analgesia of 3–5 hours have been observed with the use of the more potent, longer-acting agents such as etidocaine and bupivacaine.[130]

Table 21

LOCAL ANESTHETIC AGENTS EMPLOYED FOR INTRAVENOUS REGIONAL ANESTHESIA

Agent	Usual Conc.(%)	Usual Volume(ml) (Upper extremity)	Usual Dosage (mg/Kg)	Duration of Residual Anesthesia (min)
A. Short Duration				
PROCAINE				
CHLOROPROCAINE	0.5	20-40	1.5-3.0	30-60
B. Moderate Duration				
LIDOCAINE				
MEPIVACAINE	0.5	20-40	1.5-3.0	60-120
PRILOCAINE				
C. Long Duration				
BUPIVACAINE				
ETIDOCAINE	0.25	20-40	0.75-1.0	200-350

The concentration and volume of local anesthetic solution influences analgesic adequacy and potential safety of intravascular regional anesthesia.[168, 169, 170] In general, the use of large volumes of more dilute solutions offers the optimal conditions for satisfactory anesthesia and enhanced safety. Tucker and Boas demonstrated that the peak systemic arterial blood concentration of lidocaine following the use of a 0.5% solution was approximately 40% lower than the level observed when a 1% solution was utilized with the total dosage being equal.[170] Studies with prilocaine have shown that the peak systemic arterial blood concentration varies directly with the concentration of the anesthetic agent.[168] In general, concentrations of 0.5% lidocaine, prilocaine, or mepivacaine and 0.25% of etidocaine and bupivacaine have been utilized to produce satisfactory analgesia.[130, 163, 166] The volume of solution required depends upon the mass of tissue to be anesthetized. Thus, as stated previously, a greater volume of solution is required for procedures involving the lower limbs.

Varying dosages have been employed in intravenous regional anesthesia. Agents such as lidocaine have been administered in doses varying between 1.5 and 5 mg/kg for procedures involving the upper arm. Most commonly, 40 ml of an 0.5% solution of lidocaine (200 mg) have been found to produce satisfactory analgesia for the upper arm which would correspond to a dosage of approximately 3 mg/kg. As indicated previously, Bell, Slater, and Harris have suggested that the use of a preinjection ischemia period permits the use of a 1.5 mg/kg dosage of lidocaine with adequate analgesic effects.[162] Since larger volumes of local anesthetic solution are required for procedures involving lower limbs, the use of 75–100 ml of a dilute anesthetic solution, e.g., 0.25% lidocaine, has been advocated in order to preclude the use of excessive amounts of drug that might lead to potential adverse effects.[156, 157]

PHARMACODYNAMIC CONSIDERATIONS

Studies involving the intravascular administration of local anesthetic agents to tourniquet-occluded limbs in animals and man have shown that the drugs diffuse rapidly from the vascular compartment to the extracellular space where they are taken up by muscle and nerve.[171–173] de Jong demonstrated in cats that conduction in the small delta and C fibers was markedly reduced following intravenous regional analgesia, whereas the large alpha fibers were unaffected.[174] Studies in man have also revealed that the action potential amplitude of major nerve trunks is not significantly altered by the intravascular administration of local anesthetic drugs in a tourniquet-occluded limb.[175, 176] These studies indicate that initially the primary site of analgesic activity following intravenous regional anesthesia is at the peripheral nerve endings. However, if the dosage of anesthetic drug is increased or the period of circulatory occlusion is prolonged, conduction in major nerve trunks may be reduced.[173, 176, 177] It has also been suggested that the muscle relaxation and motor paralysis which occurs following intravenous regional analgesia may be related in part to an inhibitory effect of the local anesthetic agent on the neuromuscular junction.[175]

PERIPHERAL NERVE BLOCKADE

Regional anesthetic procedures that involve the inhibition of conduction in nerve fibers of the peripheral nervous system can be classified together under the general category of peripheral nerve blockade. This form of regional anesthesia has been subdivided arbitrarily into minor and major nerve blocks. Minor nerve blocks are defined as procedures involving single nerve entities, e.g., ulnar or radial nerve, while major nerve blocks comprise those procedures in which two or more distinct nerves or a nerve plexus are blocked, e.g., sciatic-femoral block and brachial plexus blockade.

Minor Nerve Blocks

A standardized ulnar nerve-blocking technique has been employed by Albért and Löfström to evaluate the anesthetic properties of different agents.[142, 178–181] The results obtained in these controlled human investigations agree quite well with data obtained from in vivo and in vitro animal studies. For example, a classification of the various agents according to their duration of action reveals that procaine possesses a short duration of anesthetic activity; lidocaine, mepivacaine, and prilocaine are agents of moderate duration; and tetracaine, bupivacaine, and etidocaine represent long-acting local anesthetic agents (Table 22). The duration of analgesia produced by tetracaine in these studies, however, was shorter than anticipated from clinical experience. Reappearance of pain sensation occurred in 135 minutes following the use of 0.25% tetracaine, which was significantly longer than the durations observed with the moderate acting agents, but considerably shorter than the values obtained with bupivacaine and etidocaine. Differences in anesthetic technique can

Table 22

COMPARATIVE ANESTHETIC DURATION OF LOCAL ANESTHETIC AGENTS
AS DETERMINED BY A STANDARDIZED ULNAR-BLOCK TECHNIQUE

DURATION	AGENTS	CONCENTRATION
SHORT (15 - 45 min)	PROCAINE	1.0%
MODERATE (60 - 120 min)	LIDOCAINE	1.0%
	MEPIVACAINE	1.0%
	PRILOCAINE	1.0%
LONG (400 - 450 min)	BUPIVACAINE	0.25%
	ETIDOCAINE	0.5%

markedly affect anesthetic activity. Albért and Löfström observed the reappearance of pain sensation in 40 minutes following the intraneural injections of 1 ml of 1% lidocaine, whereas Poppers and co-workers reported a duration of sensory analgesia of 165 minutes when 5 ml of this agent were administered extraneurally.[44, 179]

Dosage and concomitant use of epinephrine also can influence the activity of local anesthetic agents employed for minor nerve blocks. A significant increase in the duration of sensory analgesia and motor blockade was observed when the dose of etidocaine for ulnar nerve blocks was increased from 12.5 to 25 mg.[44] In addition, the duration of both sensory analgesia and motor blockade was prolonged significantly when epinephrine was added to various local anesthetic solutions (Fig. 4-3).[44, 80, 181] As observed in infiltration anesthesia, lidocaine appears to benefit most by the addition of epinephrine. A 200% increase in duration of sensory analgesia was produced by the addition of epinephrine to lidocaine solutions, whereas a 20% to 50% prolongation of anesthetic action occurred when a vasoconstrictor was added to agents such as mepivacaine, bupivacaine, and etidocaine.[181]

Major Nerve Blocks

It is difficult to describe in general terms the effects of local anesthetic agents on major nerve trunks or plexi, due to the marked anatomical differences involved in the blockade of major nerves. These differences are illustrated best by comparing intercostal nerve blockade with brachial plexus block. Intercostal nerve blockade usu-

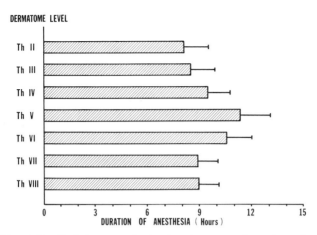

Fig. 4-5. Relative anesthetic duration at various thoracic dermatomal levels following intercostal nerve blockade with etidocaine.

ally is performed by injecting 2–4 ml of anesthetic solution around individual intercostal nerves.[182] The number of nerves to be blocked depends on the desired extent of anesthesia. In essence, this procedure consists of a series of multiple minor nerve blocks, i.e., each intercostal nerve being blocked individually. The only barriers to the neural uptake of anesthetic drug are the connective tissue and myelin sheaths of the individual intercostal nerves. An additive anesthetic effect does exist between contiguous nerves, such that the duration of anesthesia observed at the center of the area of block is significantly longer than at the peripheral dermatomal levels of the block (Fig.

Table 23

COMPARATIVE ANESTHETIC PROPERTIES OF VARIOUS AGENTS EMPLOYED
FOR MINOR AND MAJOR NERVE BLOCKS

ANESTHETIC TECHNIQUE	AGENT	CONC. (%)	VOLUME (ml)	AVERAGE ONSET TIME (min)	AVERAGE DURATION OF SENSORY ANALGESIA (min)
ULNAR NERVE BLOCK	A	1.0	1	4 - 5	60 - 120
	B	0.25 - 0.5	1	7 - 8	135 - 430
INTERCOSTAL NERVE BLOCK	A	1.0	4/nerve	3 - 5	157 - 196
	B	0.25 - 0.5	4/nerve	5 - 6	429 - 780
BRACHIAL PLEXUS BLOCK	A	1.0	40 - 50	14 - 17	195 - 245
	B	0.25 - 0.5	40 - 50	8 - 25	572 - 613

A — includes lidocaine, mepivacaine, prilocaine
B — includes bupivacaine, tetracaine, etidocaine

4-5).[183] A comparison of the anesthetic profile of intercostal nerve blockade, i.e., initial onset and total duration of analgesia, with ulnar nerve blocks and brachial plexus blockade reveals that intercostal blocks show the rapid onset of action which is characteristic of the minor nerve-blocking procedure and the long duration of analgesia which occurs following major nerve blockade (Table 23).[184, 185]

In contrast to the relative ease of depositing anesthetic drug next to intercostal nerves, it is quite difficult to inject local anesthetic agents close to the brachial plexus due to the peculiar anatomy of this region (Fig. 4-6). A "flooding" technique is frequently employed to achieve satisfactory brachial plexus blockade. This involves the use of large volumes of local anesthetic solution in order to maximize diffusion to the nerve plexus. If the solution is placed outside the connective tissue sleeve enveloping the brachial plexus, the anesthetic molecules must diffuse through several connective tissue layers surrounding the plexus. In addition, non-nervous tissue such as fat and muscle compete with the nerve trunks as depot sites for the anesthetic drug. In order to overcome such anatomical problems, various approaches to the brachial plexus have been employed such as the axillary, supraclavicular, and interscalene.[182, 186] Such technical differences can influence the analgesic results. Hollmén and Mononen reported a duration of sensory analgesia of 453 minutes when 30 ml of 0.5% etidocaine with epinephrine 1:200,000 were administered by an axillary approach,[187] whereas a duration of 572 minutes was obtained by Bromage and associates following the supraclavicular administration of the same dose of etidocaine.[188] Thus, a difference of approximately 2 hours of analgesia exists with the same

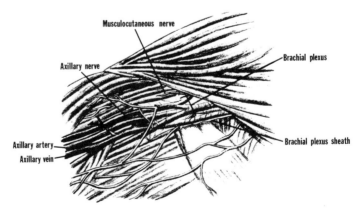

Fig. 4-6. Artist's concept of the anatomy of the axilla, with particular reference to the brachial plexus.

agent when different techniques are employed for brachial plexus blockade.

ONSET TIME

The greatest disparity between major nerve blocks, such as intercostal and brachial plexus blockade, involves the onset of anesthesia. All of the agents employed for intercostal blocks show a relatively rapid onset time, 3–6 minutes, which corresponds to the values obtained for minor nerve blocks (Table 23).[184, 185] The latency of anesthesia is considerably longer when these same drugs are used for brachial plexus or sciatic-femoral blockade (Table 23).[131, 184] In addition, a significant difference exists between the onset of various agents when brachial plexus or sciatic-femoral blocks are performed. In general, the agents of moderate duration, e.g., lidocaine and mepivacaine, exhibit a more rapid onset than the longer-acting compounds, e.g., bupivacaine and tetracaine (Table 23).[131] Bromage and Gertel have reported onset times of approximately 14 minutes for lidocaine and mepivacaine as compared to mean latency values of approximately 23 minutes for bupivacaine.[131] Etidocaine may be an exception, since the onset time of etidocaine (9 minutes) actually was shorter than that of lidocaine (14 minutes), although the duration of brachial plexus blockade with this agent (572 minutes) was similar to that of bupivacaine (575 minutes).[188]

The slow analgesic onset that characterizes major nerve-blocking procedures such as brachial plexus and sciatic-femoral blockade has been a deterrent to the use of peripheral nerve blockade for surgical procedures involving the upper and lower limbs. The onset time of agents such as lidocaine and bupivacaine can be shortened by the use of carbon dioxide salts rather than hydrochloride salts of these agents.[81, 131] Bromage and Gertel reported a reduction in the onset of brachial plexus blockade from a mean value of 14 minutes with lidocaine HCl to 8 minutes with lidocaine-CO_2.[131]

DURATION OF ANALGESIA

The longest duration of anesthesia usually occurs following major nerve blocks (Table 23). In general, the agents of moderate duration, e.g., lidocaine and mepivacaine, produce anesthesia of 1–2 hours' duration following minor nerve blockade or epidural administration, whereas analgesia usually persists for 3–4 hours when these compounds are used for major nerve blocks. Similarly, the longer-acting drugs such as tetracaine and bupivacaine cause 2–6 hours of minor nerve blockade or epidural anesthesia as compared to durations of major nerve blocks of 4–12 hours. This prolonged duration of major nerve blockade is due to several factors. In general, a greater dose of local anesthetic agent is used for major nerve blocks as compared to other types of regional anesthetic procedures (Table 23). The use of larger doses, in part, reflects an attempt to reduce onset time and also to compensate for the technical difficulties inherent in certain major nerve blocks. In addition, the region of the brachial plexus or sciatic and femoral nerves are poorly vascularized relative to other areas such as the epidural space or caudal canal. This results in a slow rate of vascular absorption of local anesthetic agents which permits a greater uptake of drug by the major nerves.[189]

The duration of major nerve blocks will be influenced by the usual factors of dosage, technique, concomitant use of vasoconstrictor agents, and basic pharmacological properties of the various local anesthetic drugs. As indicated previously, a "flooding" technique frequently is employed for procedures such as brachial plexus blockade. The use of large volumes of dilute anesthetic solutions affords a practical method of overcoming technical difficulties. However, as in other forms of regional anesthesia, total dose rather than volume or concentration of anesthetic solution appears to be the prime determinant of analgesic duration. For example, Lund and associates observed no difference in any analgesic parameter when comparing 30 ml of 0.5% etidocaine and 20 ml of 0.75% of this agent for brachial plexus blockade by the supraclavicular approach.[133]

As in infiltration anesthesia, epinephrine will prolong the duration of most local anesthetic agents employed for major nerve blocks. However, the agents of intrinsically longer duration, e.g., bupivacaine, do not benefit as much from the addition of epinephrine as do those local anesthetic drugs of short or moderate activity, e.g., procaine and lidocaine.

Although the analgesia associated with major nerve blockade persists for a longer time than in any other form of regional anesthesia, the variation in total duration of anesthesia is also considerably greater than that observed in other types of conduction blocks. This variability in anesthetic duration is particularly marked when the longer acting compounds are used for major nerve blockade. For example, the mean duration of intercostal or brachial plexus blocks is approximately 600 minutes (10 hours) for bupivacaine, but the standard deviation in both cases exceeds 100 minutes.[184] Brachial plexus blocks varying in duration from 4 to 20 hours have been reported in individual patients with the long-acting local anesthetic agents.[188] To date, no reports of irreversible major nerve blocks have appeared in the literature following the use of bupivacaine or etidocaine. It would be prudent to forewarn patients receiving these agents for major nerve-blocking procedures about the possibility of prolonged sensory and motor block in the involved region.

CENTRAL NEURAL BLOCKADE

Epidural (Peridural) Anesthesia

Anatomically, the epidural space is that area between the dura mater and the ligaments and periosteum lining the vertebral canal, extending from the foramen magnum to the sacrococcygeal membrane. This space has been described as a "potential" space, since normally it is completely filled with a loose type of adipose tissue, lymphatics, and blood vessels. It is particularly rich in venous plexi. No free fluid exists in the epidural space in contradistinction to the cerebrospinal fluid which is found in the subarachnoid space. However, solutions injected into the epidural space will spread in all directions between the loose tissue structure that occupies this area. Epidural anesthesia is usually subdivided into three categories depending on the site of injection: thoracic epidural, lumbar epidural, and caudal anesthesia. Cervical epidural anesthesia is possible but is rarely performed. Thoracic epidural anesthesia has been employed mainly for the production of a segmental band of analgesia involving the middle and lower thoracic dermatomes. This technique has proven beneficial for the relief of pain following thoracic or upper abdominal surgery. Lumbar epidural anesthesia is useful as an adjunct to surgical procedures involving the lower abdomen, pelvis, perineum, lower extremities, and obstetrical procedures. Caudal anesthesia is usually reserved for pelvic and perineal surgery and for vaginal deliveries.

MECHANISM OF EPIDURAL ANESTHESIA

The anatomy, physiology, and pharmacology of epidural anesthesia have been reviewed in an attempt to define the mechanism of this particular form of conduction blockade.[190-193] The possible sites of action of local anesthetic agents administered epidurally are the paravertebral nerve trunks, the dorsal root ganglia, the dorsal and ventral spinal roots, and the spinal cord (Fig. 4-7). Radiopaque material injected into the epidural space exits through the intervertebral foramina. It is, therefore, possible that anesthetic agents could leave

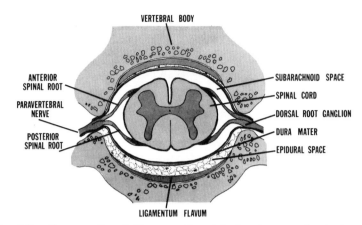

Fig. 4-7.   Cross-sectional diagram of vertebral column and spinal cord.

the epidural region via these foramina to inhibit conduction in the paravertebral nerve trunks. Under these conditions, epidural anesthesia would be analogous to multiple paravertebral blocks. However, the intervertebral foramina are patent only in young people, which might suggest a correlation between age and spread of epidural anesthesia.[194] Such a relationship has not been observed by all investigators.[195] Therefore, paravertebral blockade probably plays a minor role in the production of epidural anesthesia and, even then, only in young subjects.

The dorsal root ganglia would appear to be a logical site of action because of their anatomical location *vis à vis* the epidural space. Tissue distribution studies of local anesthetic agents administered into the subarachnoid space have revealed minimal concentrations of lidocaine in dorsal root ganglia as compared to other subdural neural structures (Fig. 4-8),[196] which suggests that dorsal-root ganglion inhibition is not a primary determinant of epidural anesthesia.

The intradural spinal roots show a high concentration of local anesthetic agent following both subarachnoid and epidural injection.[196, 197] The dermatomal progression of anesthesia following epidural administration is also consistent with conduction blockade of the spinal roots. The anatomical characteristics of the neural membranes in the region of the spinal roots favor the diffusion of anesthetic drugs. In this area, the dura mater is relatively thin, and there are numerous arachnoid villi which increase the surface area available for diffusion of anesthetic agents from the epidural space.[192] The concentration of analgesic drug localized in the dural sleeves containing the spinal roots would soon exceed the minimum effective anesthetic level required for conduction blockade of these spinal roots.

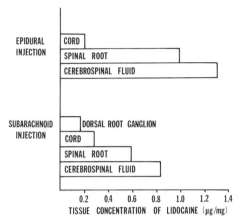

Fig. 4-8. Relative lidocaine tissue concentration following
epidural or subarachnoid injection.

The spinal cord itself also takes up anesthetic drug.[196, 197] The
concentration within the cord, however, is less than that in the spinal
roots. Moreover, a greater quantity of drug is located in the periphery
rather than the center of the cord. The dermatomal onset pattern of
epidural anesthesia and the physiological differences observed between subarachnoid and epidural anesthesia would indicate that the
spinal cord is not the initial site of action following epidural administration. However, the regression of epidural anesthesia does not
follow the same segmental distribution observed at the onset of
analgesia.[198] During the recovery phase, the cranial level of analgesia
appears as a straight line encircling the body like a belt, which would
be analogous to a transverse section through the cord. This suggests
that spinal cord blockade does occur following epidural administration of local anesthetic agents, but only after inhibition of conduction
in the spinal roots. In summary, the mechanism of epidural anesthesia
appears to be related primarily to sensory and motor spinal-root
inhibition, followed by spinal cord blockade and, possibly, in young
people, conduction block in the paravertebral nerve trunks.

FACTORS INFLUENCING QUALITY OF
EPIDURAL ANESTHESIA

Epidural anesthesia may be influenced by various factors such as
site of injection, speed of injection, patient position, patient height,
age, pregnancy, arteriosclerosis, volume and/or concentration of
anesthetic solution, and pharmacological properties of the anesthetic
agent.

Site of Injection. The dorsal epidural space is narrow from the foramen magnum to the fifth cervical vertebra. There is a gradual increase in the dorsoventral dimensions from C_5 down to the second and third lumbar vertebrae. Below this level the space again narrows.[191] Injections of small volumes of anesthetic solution (3–5 ml) into the relatively narrow midthoracic epidural space result in a discrete, but wide, segmental block. Lumbar epidural administration requires the use of larger volumes (10–30 ml) to achieve satisfactory analgesic results. Cranial spread occurs more easily than sacral spread following lumbar epidural injections, due in part to negative intrathoracic pressure and to the resistance afforded by the narrowing of the epidural space at the lumbosacral junction. A significant delay and/or an absence of analgesia at the first and second sacral segments is frequently observed following lumbar epidural injections. This has been attributed in part to the narrowing of the epidural space at the lumbosacral junction and also to the thickness of spinal roots in this region.[199] Caudal anesthesia usually requires greater amounts of drug, due to loss of solution through the anterior sacral formina and the rapid vascular absorption from this site.[189, 193, 200] Little cranial spread beyond the lumbosacral junction occurs following caudal injections because of the peculiar anatomy of the epidural space in this region.

Speed of Injection. Erdemir, Soper, and Sweet compared anesthetic qualities of 20 ml of 2% lidocaine injected into the lumbar epidural space at a rate of 1 ml/sec and 1 ml/3 sec.[201] Each of 17 subjects was studied on two occasions, so that each individual served as his own control. The slow injection resulted in a duration of motor block 10-minutes longer than achieved by the rapid injection. The level of anesthesia was approximately one dermatome higher following the fast injection. These differences were statistically significant but, obviously, are of little clinical relevance. Rate of injection had no effect on the spread of radiopaque material administered into the epidural space.[195] Probably the most pertinent clinical aspect of varying injection rate is the significantly greater patient discomfort associated with a rapid rate of injection.

Patient Position. Posture has been demonstrated by Bromage to influence the quality of epidural analgesia.[135] This investigator reported that larger quantities of anesthetic drug were required to achieve the same dermatomal level in patients in the sitting position as compared to the horizontal position. Lumbar epidural anesthesia is often performed with the patient in the sitting position in obstetrics to obtain satisfactory perineal analgesia. However, studies involving spread of radiopaque solutions and radioisotope tracers in the epidural space have failed to demonstrate any effect of posture on spread in the epidural space.[195, 202] This apparent discrepancy may be related to differences in the density of administered material. Most local anesthetic solutions are slightly hyperbaric and so would be influenced by gravity. The radiopaque and radioisotope studies may have utilized isobaric solutions, the movement of which should be independent of the influence of gravity.

Age and Height. Discrepancies also exist between studies in which the influence of age and height on epidural anesthesia has been assessed by clinical means, i.e., analgesic dermatomal levels, and by radiographic observations.[135, 194, 195] Bromage has reported that dose per segment requirements of epidurally administered analgesic agents are directly proportional to patient height and inversely proportional to patient age.[135] Burn, Guyer, and Langdon failed to demonstrate any correlation between age, height, and the spread of radiopaque material in the epidural space.[194] These authors have concluded that the degree of vertical spread in the epidural space is dependent to a greater extent on the soft tissue contents rather than the size of the epidural space and that escape of solution via the intervertebral foramina, even in young people, is of little significance.

Pregnancy. Significantly less anesthetic drug is required in pregnant patients to produce levels of epidural analgesia comparable to those in nonpregnant subjects. For example, similar epidural anesthetic results can be obtained by the use of 6–10 ml of 2% lidocaine (120–200 mg) in obstetrics and 15–30 ml of 2% lidocaine (300–600 mg) in nonparturient patients.[141, 203] This difference is believed related to inferior vena caval compression in pregnancy, which results in a marked distention of the epidural venous plexi. It is possible to mimic this situation in nonpregnant animals by placing an inflatable balloon in the inferior vena cava. Under these conditions, an exaggerated spread of epidurally administered contrast media has been observed.[204] The distended venous plexi would occupy more space, thereby decreasing the diameter of the epidural cylinder and facilitating the vertical spread of epidurally administered anesthetic solution.

Arteriosclerosis. A decrease in the dose per segment epidural requirement of local anesthetic agents has been observed in arteriosclerotic patients.[194] This is probably due to a decreased rate of vascular absorption of anesthetic agents from the epidural space by sclerotic arterioles, which allows more drug to be available for uptake by nerves. Closure of the intervertebral foramina would prevent leakage of drug through this route and also may contribute somewhat to the greater anesthetic spread in older arteriosclerotic patients.

Volume and/or Concentration of Anesthetic Solution. Much has been written about the relative influence of volume and concentration of anesthetic solutions on the quality of epidural anesthesia. Volume will influence the vertical spread of epidural analgesia.[201] For example, 30 ml of 1% lidocaine produced a level of analgesia following lumbar epidural administration, which was 4.3 dermatomes higher than that achieved by 10 ml of 3% lidocaine.[201] However, the essential qualities of epidural anesthesia, i.e., onset, depth, and duration of sensory analgesia and motor blockade are related to the mass of drug (total mg), rather than variations in volume or concentration of solution (Fig. 4-2).[141, 193] Since the primary mechanism of epidural anesthesia involves spinal root blockade, the main anesthetic determinant would be the transdural drug gradient which, in turn, is a function of the epidural drug mass, i.e., the product of volume times concentration.

Anesthetic Agent. The basic pharmacological properties of the various local anesthetic agents will influence the dosage requirements and resultant quality of epidural anesthesia. The drugs utilized for epidural anesthesia may be classified according to their intrinsic anesthetic potency and duration of action (Table 24). Procaine, chloroprocaine, lidocaine, mepivacaine, and prilocaine are commonly administered as 1% to 3% solutions, whereas tetracaine, bupivacaine, and etidocaine are employed in concentrations of 0.25% to 1.5%. These agents can be divided into three categories based on analgesic duration: short action (30–90 minutes), e.g., procaine and chloroprocaine; moderate duration (60–180 minutes), e.g., lidocaine, mepivacaine, and prilocaine; long duration (180–360 minutes), e.g., tetracaine, bupivacaine, and etidocaine.[140, 205]

Onset of epidural anesthesia may be separated into initial onset, i.e., the time at which analgesia to pin prick is observed at any dermatomal level, and complete onset, i.e., the time required for maximal segmental spread of analgesia. Initial onset usually occurs within 5–10 minutes following epidural administration of the various agents. Complete onset commonly occurs at 10–20 minutes after

Table 24

COMPARISON OF LOCAL ANESTHETIC AGENTS EMPLOYED IN EPIDURAL ANESTHESIA

AGENT	USUAL CONC. (%)	USUAL VOL. (ml)	TOTAL DOSE* (mg)	DURATION (min)
A. Short Duration				
PROCAINE	1 - 2	15 - 30	150 - 600	30 - 90
CHLOROPROCAINE	1 - 3	15 - 30	150 - 900	
B. Moderate Duration				
LIDOCAINE	1 - 2	15 - 30	150 - 500	
MEPIVACAINE	1 - 2	15 - 30	150 - 500	60 - 180
PRILOCAINE	1 - 3	15 - 30	150 - 600	
C. Long Duration				
TETRACAINE	0.25 - 0.5	15 - 30	37.5 - 150	
BUPIVACAINE	0.25 - 0.75	15 - 30	37.5 - 225	180 - 360
ETIDOCAINE	1 - 1.5	15 - 30	150 - 300	

* doses of epinephrine-containing solutions

injection of the anesthetic solution. Differences in epidural onset time between the various agents are significantly less than observed following other regional anesthetic techniques such as brachial plexus blockade (Table 25). For example, an average difference of approximately 10 minutes in onset time was observed between mepivacaine and bupivacaine in brachial plexus blocks, whereas an average difference of only 1.5 minutes existed when these agents were used for epidural anesthesia.[131] Marked variations in onset of epidural anesthesia have been reported by various investigators studying the same agent. Such variations are probably related to the method of evaluation (Table 26).[132, 134, 207–210]

Table 25

COMPARATIVE ONSET TIMES AND ANALGESIC DURATIONS OF VARIOUS LOCAL ANESTHETIC AGENTS IN BRACHIAL PLEXUS BLOCKADE AND EPIDURAL ANESTHESIA**

ANESTHETIC TECHNIQUE	ANESTHETIC AGENT	USUAL CONC.(%)	AVERAGE ONSET TIME (min ± S.E.)	AVERAGE ANALGESIC DURATION (min ± S.E.)
BRACHIAL PLEXUS BLOCK 40 - 50 ml	LIDOCAINE	1.0	14.04 ± 3.83	195 ± 26.3
	MEPIVACAINE	1.0	14.84 ± 6.22	245 ± 26.8
	BUPIVACAINE	0.25	23.26 ± 7.93	575
	ETIDOCAINE	0.5	8.77	572
EPIDURAL ANESTHESIA 20 - 30 ml	LIDOCAINE	2.0	15	100 ± 20 *
	MEPIVACAINE	2.0	15	115 ± 15
	BUPIVACAINE	0.5	16.5	195 ± 30
	ETIDOCAINE	1.0	10.85	170 ± 57

* 2-segment regression
** Data derived from ref. 128, 185

Table 26

COMPARATIVE EVALUATION BY VARIOUS INVESTIGATORS OF THE ANESTHETIC PROPERTIES OF
0.5% BUPIVACAINE WITH EPINEPHRINE 1:200,000 IN EPIDURAL ANESTHESIA

INVESTIGATOR (REFERENCE NO.)	EVALUATION TECHNIQUE	INITIAL ONSET	COMPLETE ONSET	2 SEGMENT REGRESSION	TOTAL REGRESSION
132	PIN PRICK	6.3±1.2	—	228 ± 23	—
134	PIN PRICK	9.0±1.0	18.0±2.0	160 ± 20	315±22
188	PIN PRICK	5.8	18.2	196 ± 31	—
206	TIME OF POST-OP PAIN	—	—	—	423±15
207	PIN PRICK POST-OP PAIN	12.2±1.1	28.3±2.03	—	261±23
208	PIN PRICK	7	21	210	330
209	ALLIS CLAMP	5.4±1.7	19.6±5.5	332± 169	459±82
210	PIN PRICK	9.2±4.0	19.8±6.2	156 ± 68	284±111

Analgesic duration is commonly divided into (a) 2-segment regression, i.e., the time required for analgesia to regress 2 dermatomes
from the highest level of block, and (b) total duration, i.e., the time
for complete disappearance of analgesia from all dermatomes. The
time interval between 2-segment regression and total recovery from
analgesia is considerably longer for the long-acting agents as compared to the agents of moderate total duration (Fig. 4-9).[211] In general, the duration of epidural anesthesia is markedly shorter than the
duration of major nerve blockade. However, the difference in duration between epidural and major nerve blockade is less for agents
such as lidocaine and mepivacaine than for those compounds possessing an intrinsically longer duration of action, e.g., bupivacaine and

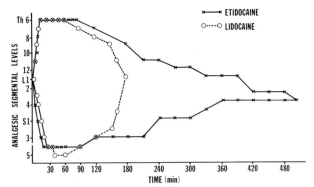

Fig. 4-9. Comparative   time-segment   diagrams   for
lidocaine and etidocaine following epidural administration.

tetracaine (Table 25). Considerable variation also exists in the values for anesthetic duration reported by different investigators for the same agent, which again reflects differences in the method of analgesic evaluation (Table 26).[132, 134, 206-210]

Duration of anesthesia may be influenced by the concomitant use of vasoconstrictor agents. In general, the duration of agents of short or moderate activity is significantly prolonged by the use of epinephrine-containing solutions, whereas the long-acting agents benefit little from the addition of epinephrine.[141, 145, 209] The optimal concentration of epinephrine required to retard the vascular absorption of local anesthetic agents from the epidural space and so prolong the duration of anesthesia may vary depending on the relative vasodilator properties of the different analgesic drugs. The optimal concentration of epinephrine for each anesthetic agent has not been well elucidated. A 1:200,000 (5 μg/ml) concentration of epinephrine usually is employed with all epidurally administered anesthetic drugs. This concentration of epinephrine has been demonstrated to be optimal for lidocaine and etidocaine.[212, 213]

With regard to the use of other vasoconstrictor agents, phenylephrine has been compared with epinephrine as an additive to solutions of lidocaine for epidural anesthesia.[214] A concentration of 50 μg/ml (1:20,000) of phenylephrine added to 2% lidocaine produced a duration of epidural analgesia which was approximately 45 minutes shorter than that achieved by a 2% lidocaine solution with epinephrine 1:200,000 (5 μg/ml). This shorter analgesic duration of the lidocaine-phenylephrine solution was correlated with a higher peak blood level of lidocaine, which suggests that the vasoconstrictor effect of phenylephrine was not comparable to that of epinephrine at the concentrations studied.

Epidural anesthesia has proven to be a useful technique for differential nerve blockade and for unmasking subtle differences between agents that are not seen in other forms of regional anesthesia. As indicated previously, nerve fibers have been classified according to their conduction velocity as A, B, and C fibers (Table 27).[215] The A fibers are further subdivided into alpha, beta, gamma, and delta in order of decreasing conduction velocity. A fibers consist of both sensory- and motor-myelinated fibers. The A delta fibers are believed responsible for fast pain sensation. B fibers are found in myelinated preganglionic autonomic nerves. C fibers consist of unmyelinated sensory and postganglionic autonomic fibers. In general, the conduction velocity of these different fibers is directly proportional to their size, i.e., the fast-conducting A fibers are largest, whereas the slow-conducting C fibers are smallest. It appears that the size of the nerve fibers influences the minimum anesthetic concentration required for conduction block, i.e., the larger fibers have a higher Cm. On the basis of this anatomical and physiological knowledge, it is possible to administer varying doses of local anesthetic agents epidurally in order to selectively block different nerve fibers. For example, sympathetic nerve blockade may be performed with 5–7 ml of 0.5% to 1.0% lidocaine or mepivacaine, whereas 15–20 ml of 1% to 2% solutions are required for complete sensory and motor block.[182] The onset and duration of sympathetic, sensory, and motor block differ following epidural anesthesia. The onset of sympathetic and sensory block occurs most rapidly, followed by motor blockade, while regression occurs in the opposite direction, i.e., motor function returns initially, followed by sensory and sympathetic activity (Table 27). Sympathetic block following epidural administration of local anesthetic drugs mainly involves inhibition of the preganglionic sympathetic B fibers. The A delta fibers conduct rapid and sharp pain impulses and, due to their larger size and higher Cm requirements, may become unblocked sooner than B fibers. Thus, sensory activity may return sooner than sympathetic tone. Hypotension may occur if patients are ambulated too soon following epidural anesthesia, in the mistaken impression that sympathetic activity has fully returned when sensation appears completely recovered.[216]

An interrelationship exists between the anatomy of the epidural space, the morphology of nerve fibers involved in epidural anesthesia, and the physicochemical properties of the local anesthetic agents employed for this procedure. This is best exemplified by comparing the epidural anesthetic results obtained with bupivacaine and

Table 27

CLASSIFICATION OF NERVE FIBERS ACCORDING TO ANATOMICAL AND PHYSIOLOGICAL PROPERTIES

CLASS	DIAMETER (microns)	MYELINATED	FUNCTION	CONDUCTION VELOCITY (m/sec)	C_m	ORDER OF BLOCK	ORDER OF RECOVERY
A Fibers	2-22	+		10-120	HIGHEST	3	1
α			MOTOR				
β			MOTOR				
γ			MOTOR				
δ			SENSORY				
B Fibers	1-3	+	PREGANGLIONIC AUTONOMIC	10-20	INTERMEDIATE	2	2
C Fibers	0.5-1	−	SENSORY POSTGANGLIONIC AUTONOMIC	0.5-2.0	LOWEST	1	3

etidocaine. These two agents possess the same intrinsic anesthetic potency as determined on an isolated nerve.[114, 115] However, in the epidural space of man, a 1% concentration of etidocaine is equivalent to 0.5% bupivacaine in terms of sensory blockade.[210] This difference is probably attributable to the very high lipid solubility of etidocaine which results in an uptake and sequestration of this compound by the extensive adipose tissue in the epidural space. The high lipid solubility and lower pK_a of etidocaine are probably responsible for the rapid diffusion of this agent through the dura and myelin covering of A fibers, which leads to a more rapid onset of motor blockade.[210] Moreover, the profoundness and longer duration of motor block observed with etidocaine suggests an accumulation in the lipid myelin sheaths of the A fibers.[188, 210]

Spinal Anesthesia

This form of regional anesthesia represents the oldest and still the most commonly employed type of central neural blockade. This procedure was described in the last decade of the nineteenth century by Halsted and his associates and by August Bier. In recent years, this form of central neural blockade has been the subject of much controversy related, particularly, to the potential hazards and complications associated with spinal anesthesia. Several studies of a prospective and retrospective nature have been published in which the hazards of subarachnoid blockade have been evaluated.[217-220] Noble and Murray reviewed the experiences of 27 Canadian university-affiliated hospitals in which a total of 78,746 spinal anesthetic procedures had been conducted between the years of 1959 and 1969.[221] These authors concluded that the hazards of spinal block are no greater than that of any other anesthetic technique and that the procedure should be retained as part of the armamentarium of the anesthesiologist.

COMPARISON OF EPIDURAL AND
SPINAL ANESTHESIA

Moore and co-workers compared both forms of central neural blockade involving approximately 20,000 patients and stated that both these techniques are safe, provided the physician performing the procedure evaluates his own capabilities and the patient's physical status.[222] The anesthetic characteristics of subdural and extradural procedures differ somewhat (Table 28). The onset time for subarachnoid blocks is appreciably shorter than that observed following

Table 28

COMPARISON OF SPINAL AND EPIDURAL ANESTHESIA

PROCEDURE	AGENTS*	USUAL CONC.(%)	USUAL VOL(ml)	TOTAL DOSE (mg)	TONICITY RELATIVE to CSF	GLUCOSE CONC.	COMPLETE ONSET (min)	DURATION (min)
SPINAL ANESTHESIA	LIDOCAINE	1.5,5.0	1-2	15-100	hyperbaric	7.5%	3-6	30-90
more controllable more predictable less segmental	TETRACAINE	0.25, 0.5, 1.0	1-4	5-20	isobaric hypobaric hyperbaric	5% (hyperbaric sol'n only)	5-12	75-150
EPIDURAL ANESTHESIA	LIDOCAINE	1.0,1.5,2.0	10-30	100-300	isobaric	—	10-20	45-120
less controllable less predictable more segmental	TETRACAINE	0.25,0.5	10-30	25-150	isobaric	—	15-25	120-240

*values are based on anesthetic solutions without epinephrine

epidural administration. Moore and associates reported an average onset time of 5–12 minutes for spinal block as compared to 15–25 minutes for epidural anesthesia.[222] Other investigators have reported an immediate onset with agents such as lidocaine and mepivacaine administered into the subarachnoid space.[223, 224] The more rapid onset of spinal anesthesia is understandable, since minimal diffusion barriers exist in the subarachnoid space. This lack of a diffusion barrier is readily apparent when the biotoxin substances, tetrodotoxin and saxitoxin, are employed for regional anesthesia. In the subarachnoid space, the biotoxins show a rapid onset of action and a high frequency of satisfactory analgesia. However, when these agents are administered extradurally either for epidural anesthesia or for peripheral nerve blocks in animals, the onset of anesthesia is extremely prolonged, and, generally, the incidence of satisfactory analgesia is very poor.

The duration of spinal anesthesia is generally shorter than that of epidural anesthesia. For example, an average duration of spinal anesthesia of 156–190 minutes has been reported for tetracaine as compared to a value of 334 minutes when this agent was used for epidural analgesia.[225] This difference in duration is probably due, in part, to the smaller total dosage of drug employed for spinal anesthesia as compared to epidural anesthesia (Table 28).

The area of anesthesia produced by spinal blockade is more predictable, controllable, and less segmental than that obtained with epidural administration of analgesic drugs.[222] The use of anesthetic solutions of varying tonicity and the ease of altering anesthetic level by patient posture accounts for the greater predictability and controllability of spinal anesthesia. The uptake of larger amounts of anesthetic drug by the spinal cord probably is responsible for the absence of a segmental pattern of anesthesia following subarachnoid injection.

FACTORS AFFECTING SPINAL ANESTHESIA

The analgesic properties of subarachnoid blockade may be influenced by a number of factors that can be related to the patient, anesthetic solution, and anesthetic technique.

Patient Factors. Patient position during and immediately following subdural administration of a local anesthetic agent will influence the spread of spinal anesthesia.[226] Since hyperbaric anesthetic solutions are commonly used for subarachnoid blocks, the spread in cerebrospinal fluid will be affected by gravity. For example, the patient in a sitting position at the time of injection will experience a lower level block than the patient who is supine.

A decrease in the spinal fluid capacity of the subarachnoid space will markedly affect the degree of analgesia and the dose requirements for satisfactory spinal anesthesia. Inferior vena cava compression, usually due to pregnancy, is the most common cause of engorgement and distention of the vertebral system, which will decrease the capacity of the subarachnoid space for spinal fluid. Subarachnoid administration of 4 mg of tetracaine usually produces analgesia to the T_{11} dermatomal level in normal subjects. This same dose of tetracaine will result in a T_{7-8} level of anesthesia in pregnant patients or subjects in whom inferior vena cava pressure has been experimentally elevated by abdominal compression.[227] These data support the general clinical impression that the dosage requirements for spinal anesthesia are significantly lower in pregnant patients than in nonparturient subjects.

Anesthetic Factors. Although most anesthetic drugs may be used for spinal anesthesia,[226] essentially only two agents are prepared in a form specifically intended for subarachnoid administration. Lidocaine is available as a hyperbaric solution in concentrations of 1.5% and 5.0% with 7.5% glucose. Tetracaine, which is the most commonly used spinal agent, is available both as niphanoid crystals and as a 1% solution which may be diluted with 10% glucose to obtain a 0.25% or 0.5% hyperbaric tetracaine solution. Hypobaric and isobaric solutions of tetracaine also have been utilized for specific operative situations, e.g., anorectal or hip surgery in which it may be advantageous to maintain the patient in a head-down position.[228, 229]

Lidocaine essentially provides a short duration of spinal anesthesia, whereas tetracaine is considered to be an agent of long duration. An average total analgesic duration of 94 minutes has been reported following the use of 1 ml of 5% lidocaine (50 mg)[130] with variations in duration of 30 to 150 minutes when doses of 50–250 mg are employed.[223, 230] However, surgical anesthesia for 30 to 75 minutes is usually obtained with the routine use of 1–2 ml of 5% lidocaine (50–100 mg). Tetracaine in doses of 4–20 mg has been reported to provide 75 to 105 minutes of surgical anesthesia for intraabdominal procedures and 120 to 150 minutes of surgical anesthesia for perineal and lower-extremity procedures.[222]

As in other forms of regional anesthesia, vasoconstrictor agents may prolong the duration of spinal anesthesia. The addition of 0.25–0.3 mg of epinephrine to lidocaine or tetracaine solutions will produce a 50% prolongation of spinal anesthesia.[223, 231] Measurements of spinal fluid concentrations of lidocaine following subarachnoid administration have revealed that epinephrine slows the rate of disappearance of anesthetic drug from spinal fluid, probably because of its vasoconstrictor effects.[223] An increase in the duration of subarachnoid block has also been reported following the addition of 5 mg of phenylephrine to tetracaine.[231]

Technical Factors. The site of injection will influence the analgesic dermatomal level. The L_{3-4} interspace is commonly used for the subarachnoid administration of anesthetic drugs. Injection at higher vertebral interspaces is associated with a higher level of block. The speed of injection, needle direction, and type of spinal needle may influence the level of spinal anesthesia.[225] Use of a unidirectional needle positioned in a cephalad direction will produce a higher level of sensory analgesia. Injection of tetracaine at a rate of 1 ml/sec produced a level of analgesia which was approximately 2 dermatomal levels higher than was achieved with an injection rate of 0.2 ml/sec. Moreover, the use of a unidirectional needle resulted in a higher analgesic level than that obtained with a conventional needle, regardless of injection rate.[225]

TACHYPHYLAXIS

The continuous infusion or intermittent injection of local anesthetic agents into the epidural or subdural space has been employed for prolonged surgical procedures or to provide an extended period of postoperative pain relief. However, tachyphylaxis, or rapid tolerance, has been observed to occur following the continuous or repeated administration of local anesthetic agents into the subarachnoid or epidural space.[232-234] Tachyphylaxis is defined as a rapidly developing decreased analgesic response to a constant repeated dose of a specific local anesthetic drug. Bromage and associates have carefully described the development of tachyphylaxis in a group of patients undergoing epidural anesthesia.[233] A progressive decrease in duration and spread of anesthesia was observed as the interval between the return of sensation and the subsequent injection was increased from 10 to 60 minutes, reaching a constant degree of tachyphylaxis when the interanalgesic interval exceeded 60 minutes. A constant 30% reduction in response to each successive injection occurred at maximum tolerance.

The etiology of local anesthetic tachyphylaxis has not been completely resolved. Cohen and associates have proposed that the development of tolerance following repetitive subarachnoid administration is related to changes in the pH of cerebrospinal fluid (CSF).[234] A significant increase in the H^+ content of CSF was observed when multiple subarachnoid injections of acidic solutions of lidocaine and procaine were made. This greater H^+ content (lower pH) of CSF would tend to increase the amount of the ionized form of a local anesthetic agent and conversely produce a relative decrease in the base form, which is responsible for diffusion through the nerve membrane. Such an alteration would be manifested clinically as a reduced analgesic response. Consistent with this hypothesis was the observation that a correlation existed between the rate of development of tachyphylaxis and the pK_a of the local anesthetic agent. For example, tolerance occurred more rapidly when an agent with a lower pK_a, e.g., mepivacaine was used. The relative proportion of base and cationic form of such a drug would be affected to a greater degree by alterations in the pH of CSF than would an agent with a higher pK_a. These studies suggest that the development of tachyphylaxis may be retarded by the use of agents with intrinsically longer durations of action, use of agents with higher pK_a values, and use of a buffer to prevent the decrease in pH of cerebrospinal fluid.

TOPICAL ANESTHESIA

Topical anesthesia is an extremely complex subject, due to a number of complicating factors such as lack of reliable objective techniques for evaluating anesthetic activity, variability in application site, and diversity of anesthetic application forms.[235]

Site of Application

Anesthetic agents have been applied topically to such diverse sites as skin, eye, tympanic membrane of the ear, gastrointestinal tract, gingival mucosa, tracheobronchial tree, genitourinary tract, and rectum. Endotracheal instillation of local anesthetic agents for endoscopy and bronchoscopy represents one of the most common uses of topical anesthesia.[236] Cocaine, tetracaine, lidocaine, and prilocaine have been reported to be efficacious for topical anesthesia of the oropharynx, larynx, and tracheobronchial tree.[237-239] Onset of anesthesia usually occurs in 5–10 minutes, and analgesic duration as judged by suppression of the cough reflex persists for approximately 30 minutes with lidocaine and prilocaine.[239] The duration of cocaine and tetracaine probably averages 60 minutes, although definitive values based on control studies are lacking.

Attempts have been made to utilize local anesthetic drugs orally for the treatment of conditions such as peptic esophagitis and duodenal ulcers.[240, 241] The rationale for the oral use of local anesthetic agents is the ability to inhibit the formation or release of gastrin by a blockade of vagal nerve endings. The extremely low gastric pH renders most of the conventional local anesthetic agents orally ineffective. However, oxethazaine was introduced as a local anesthetic compound that was active in a low pH environment.[242] Oxethazaine has been reported to be effective for the treatment of peptic esophagitis and duodenal ulcers,[240, 241] but it has not been possible to demonstrate a gastrin inhibitory effect with the drug.[243]

Topical anesthesia is frequently employed as an adjunct to various diagnostic urologic procedures to obviate the need for general anesthesia. The urethral instillation of lidocaine incorporated in a highly viscid gel has been demonstrated to produce a significant increase in pain threshold as evaluated by an electrical stimulation technique.[244]

Mucous membranes such as the gingiva are a common site for the application of topical anesthetic agents. Adriani and associates have conducted a series of studies to determine the topical anesthetic properties of various drugs on mucous membranes and the factors which influence their action.[245-248] A standardized technique involving electrical stimulation of the tip of the tongue was utilized to evaluate over 40 drugs. Tetracaine, cocaine, dibucaine, lidocaine, and dyclonine were found to be the most potent and effective topical anesthetic agents.[246, 247] Marked differences were found in the anesthetic properties of different agents when topical administration was compared to administration by injection. For example, tetracaine and

Table 29

COMPARATIVE TOPICAL AND INJECTABLE ANESTHETIC ACTIVITY
OF VARIOUS LOCAL ANESTHETIC AGENTS

AGENT	EFFECTIVE ANESTHETIC CONCENTRATIONS	
	INJECTABLE	TOPICAL
PROCAINE	1.0 – 4.0%	10 – 20%
TETRACAINE	0.25 – 1.0%	0.2 – 1.0%
LIDOCAINE	0.5 – 2.0%	2.0 – 4.0%
MEPIVACAINE	0.5 – 2.0%	12 – 15%

lidocaine provide effective anesthesia by surface application and local injection, whereas procaine and mepivacaine are very effective anesthetic agents when administered by injection, but display poor topical anesthetic properties (Table 29).

An increase in dose will shorten the onset and prolong the duration of surface anesthesia as observed in other forms of regional anesthesia (Fig. 4-10). The onset of anesthesia with cocaine is reduced from 4 to 0.3

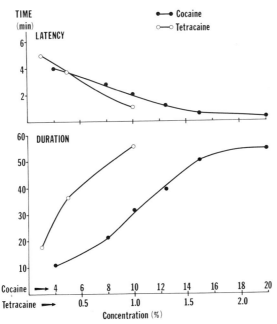

Fig. 4-10.   Effect of anesthetic concentration on the onset and duration of topical analgesia.

minutes and the duration prolonged from 10 to 55 minutes as the cocaine concentration is increased from 4 to 20%. The addition of vasoconstrictor drugs, colloids, detergents, cations, and spreading agents did not influence either the intensity or duration of topical anesthesia.[246, 247]

The topical application of local anesthetic agents to intact skin generally fails to produce a measurable degree of cutaneous analgesia unless high concentrations of certain compounds are maintained in contact with the skin for relatively long periods of time (30–60 minutes). Twenty percent benzocaine and 30–40% lidocaine have been reported to produce anesthesia of intact skin.[249, 250] In the case of lidocaine, the use of an occlusive bandage to ensure cutaneous contact for approximately 60 minutes was required to demonstrate surface analgesia. Thus, the onset of anesthesia is slow and the duration and depth of anesthesia is marginal. The lack of cutaneous efficacy may be related either to an inability of the presently available agents to penetrate the epithelial barriers of intact skin or to a rapid vascular absorption following diffusion through the epidermis such that insufficient drug is taken up by the nerve endings in the dermis.

TOPICAL ANESTHETIC APPLICATION FORMS

The composition of topical anesthetic preparations varies markedly, depending on the intended site of application (Table 30). For example, lidocaine is prepared in the following forms for topical use: a 4% aqueous solution for endotracheal instillation; a 2.5–5.0% ointment containing polyethylene and propylene glycol for anesthesia of mucous membranes; a 2% jelly containing carboxymethylcellulose for intraurethral use; a suppository of 100 mg lidocaine for rectal application, and a 10% aerosol for anesthesia of the gingival mucosa. Other agents such as tetracaine, benzocaine, and dibucaine are also prepared in various forms for topical anesthesia. The comparative efficacy of various application forms has been evaluated by means of an electrical stimulating device attached to the gingival mucosa. Giddon and co-workers reported that lidocaine incorporated into a dissolvable film produced a significantly greater increase in pain threshold than the same dose of lidocaine applied either in the form of an ointment, liquid, or spray.[251] The main purpose of these various topical admixtures is to maintain the anesthetic agent in contact with the surface intended to be anesthetized. The various ingredients in the topical anesthetic preparation are not believed to enhance the basic conduction-blocking properties of the anesthetic drug.

Table 30

VARIOUS PREPARATIONS INTENDED FOR TOPICAL ANESTHESIA

ANESTHETIC INGREDIENT	CONCENTRATION %	PHARMACEUTICAL APPLICATION FORM	INTENDED AREA OF USE
BENZOCAINE	1·5	Cream	Skin and mucous membrane
	20	Ointment	Skin and mucous membrane
	20	Aerosol	Skin and mucous membrane
COCAINE	4	Solution	Ear, nose, throat
DIBUCAINE	0.25·1	Cream	Skin
	0.25·1	Ointment	Skin
	0.25·1	Aerosol	Skin
	0.25	Solution	Ear
	2.5	Suppositories	Rectum
DYCLONINE	0.5·1	Solution	Skin, oro-pharynx, tracheo-bronchial tree, urethra, rectum
LIDOCAINE	2·4	Solution	Oro-pharynx, tracheobronchial tree, nose
	2	Jelly	Urethra
	2.5·5	Ointment	Skin, mucous membrane, rectum
	2	Viscous	Oro-pharynx
	10	Suppositories	Rectum
	10	Aerosol	Gingival mucosa
TETRACAINE	0.5·1	Ointment	Skin, rectum, mucous membrane
	0.5·1	Cream	Skin, rectum, mucous membrane
	0.25·1	Solution	Nose, tracheobronchial tree

SUMMARY

1. Local anesthetic activity varies as a function of the regional anesthetic procedure, clinical status of the patient, anesthetic agent, and composition of anesthetic solution.

2. Regional anesthesia may be classified anatomically as follows: (a) infiltration anesthesia (extravascular or intravascular); (b) peripheral nerve blockade (minor or major nerve block); (c) central neural blockade (epidural or subarachnoid block); and (d) topical anesthesia.

3. In general, onset of anesthesia occurs most rapidly during infiltration techniques and subarachnoid administration followed in order of increasing onset time by minor nerve blockade, epidural block, and topical application to mucous membranes. The longest latency is observed in peripheral nerve blockade involving major nerve trunks and plexi. Duration of anesthesia is most prolonged when major nerve blockade is performed, followed in order of decreasing duration by epidural and infiltration procedures, minor nerve and subarachnoid blocks, and topical application.

4. The local anesthetic agents commonly employed for regional

anesthesia may be classified according to their relative duration of activity; agents of short duration, e.g., procaine and chloroprocaine; agents of moderate duration, e.g., lidocaine, mepivacaine, and prilocaine; and agents of long duration, e.g., tetracaine, bupivacaine, and etidocaine.

5. In general, the onset, duration, and quality of regional anesthesia are enhanced by an increase in dose achieved either by an increase in concentration or volume of anesthetic solution and by the concomitant use of a vasoconstrictor drug, epinephrine. However, the local anesthetic properties of the intrinsically more potent and longer-acting agents are influenced less by the addition of epinephrine, particularly when such agents are employed for central neural blockade of the epidural type.

6. The properties of topical anesthesia are influenced by the site of application, the pharmaceutical administration form, and the local anesthetic agent. Tetracaine, cocaine, dibucaine, benzocaine, dyclonine, lidocaine, and prilocaine demonstrate effective topical anesthetic activity, whereas procaine and mepivacaine provide weak surface anesthesia. Intact skin is generally resistant to the anesthetic effect of the conventional agents.

5
Pharmacokinetic Aspects of Local Anesthetic Agents

Local anesthetic agents are applied directly to the region of the body in which they exert their desired pharmacological action, whereas other therapeutic agents usually are administered either parenterally or orally and then transported by the circulatory system to their target organ, located at some distance from the site of administration. Local anesthetic activity and, particularly, the toxicity of this class of drugs are influenced by factors such as systemic absorption from site of injection, distribution, metabolism, and excretion. Due in large part to the development of specific and sensitive analytical methods, such as gas chromatography, for measuring the concentration of local anesthetic drugs in blood and urine, a considerable body of information is presently available concerning the physiological disposition of local anesthetic agents.

ABSORPTION

The most important determinants of absorption are (a) the site of injection, (b) the dosage of local anesthetic agent administered, (c) the addition of a vasoconstrictor agent to the local anesthetic solution, and (d) the pharmacological profile of the local anesthetic drug itself (Table 31).[143,189,212]

Site of Injection
The blood levels of different local anesthetic agents have been measured following their administration into various anatomical sites. In general, a consistent pattern of vascular absorption exists regard-

Table 31

FACTORS INFLUENCING ABSORPTION OF LOCAL
ANESTHETIC AGENTS

1. SITE OF INJECTION

2. DOSAGE

3. ADDITION OF A VASOCONSTRICTOR AGENT

4. PHARMACOLOGICAL CHARACTERISTICS OF DRUG

less of the anesthetic agent employed; namely, (a) the highest anesthetic blood level is obtained following intercostal nerve blockade, [143, 189, 212] (b) the maximum concentration of local analgesic agent in blood decreases according to the site of administration in the following order: caudal canal, lumbar epidural space, brachial plexus region, and sciatic-femoral region, [143, 189, 200, 212] (c) the lowest anesthetic blood levels have been observed following subcutaneous administration of local anesthetic agents for infiltration anesthesia [143, 252] (Fig. 5-1). This general pattern of systemic absorption from various sites of administration has been demonstrated for lidocaine, prilocaine, mepivacaine, and etidocaine[143,185,189,212] (Fig. 5-1). The fact that anesthetic blood levels differ following administration into different anatomical sites is related to a multiplicity of factors. The high blood concentration observed following intercostal nerve blockade is probably attributable to the multiple injections required for this peripheral nerve-blocking procedure such that the local anesthetic solution is exposed to a larger vascular surface area, which results in a greater rate and degree of absorption. The higher anesthetic blood levels obtained following caudal anesthesia as compared to lumbar epidural administration may reflect the greater vascularity of the bony tissue in the caudal canal, which could promote the systemic absorption of local anesthetic agents from that site.[253] In addition, there are relatively large amounts of adipose tissue in the lumbar epidural space, which could serve as a depot site for local anesthetic agents, thereby tending to retard vascular absorption.[200, 212] An interesting study comparing anesthetic blood levels following different modes of administration was conducted by Mazze and Dunbar.[161] The venous blood levels of lidocaine were determined after brachial plexus blockade and intravenous regional anesthesia to evaluate the relative safety of these regional anesthetic techniques for certain surgical procedures involving the upper limb. A significantly lower

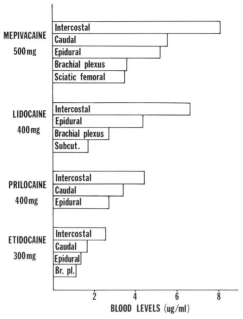

Fig. 5-1. Comparative peak blood levels of several local anesthetic agents following administration into various anatomical sites.

venous blood level of lidocaine was observed following tourniquet release in the intravenous regional procedure (1.5 ± 0.2 μg/ml) as compared to the peak lidocaine blood level after brachial plexus blockade (2.5 ± 0.5 μg/ml). This relationship of administration site to rate of drug absorption has obvious clinical significance, since the same dose of a local anesthetic agent may be potentially toxic in one injection area, but not in others. For example, average peak blood levels in excess of 6 μg/ml have been reported with the use of 400 to 500 mg of lidocaine and mepivacaine for intercostal nerve blockade, as compared to average peak blood levels of 4–5 μg/ml when the same dose of these two drugs was employed for lumbar epidural anesthesia. [143, 189] Since the frequency of adverse events is greater when the blood level of lidocaine and mepivacaine exceeds 5 μg/ml, the results of these studies would indicate that the potential for systemic local anesthetic toxicity is significantly greater following intercostal nerve blockade than after lumbar epidural anesthesia, despite the use of the same total dose of local anesthetic agent for both procedures.

Absorption of local anesthetic agents is affected not only by administration into markedly different anatomical sites, but also by injection into different muscle masses (Fig. 5-2). A significantly higher peak blood level has been observed to occur following administration of lidocaine into the deltoid muscle as compared to injection into the vastus lateralis and gluteus maximus.[254-256] The greater absorption from the deltoid muscle appears related to the greater blood flow in that particular muscle mass than in the vastus lateralis.[257] The extremely low levels of lidocaine following injection into the gluteus maximus may reflect the greater adiposity in this region which could serve as a depot site for the local anesthetic agent and so retard its vascular absorption. Again, this variation in absorption from different muscle sites has practical clinical applicability. In this particular situation, the use of different muscle sites has therapeutic rather than toxic implications when a drug such as lidocaine is used for antiarrhythmic purposes. Thus, 200–300 mg of lidocaine injected into the deltoid muscle produces a blood level in excess of 2 μg/ml, which is normally considered to be adequate for antiarrhythmic activity. This same dose of lidocaine injected into the gluteus maximus or vastus lateralis results in a peak venous blood level of less than 2 μg/ml, which is usually inadequate for antiarrhythmic therapy[256] (Fig. 5-3).

The topical application of local anesthetic agents at various sites also results in differences in absorption and toxicity[124] (Fig. 5-4). In general, the rate of absorption of local anesthetic agents occurs most rapidly following intratracheal administration. The relative absorption

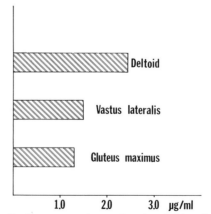

Fig. 5-2. Peak venous plasma levels of lidocaine following administration into different muscle sites.

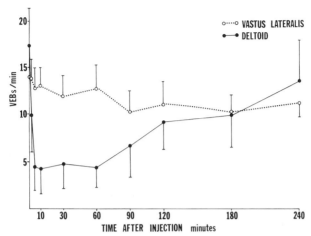

Fig. 5-3. Frequency of ventricular extrasystoles (VEB) following intramuscular administration of 300 mg lidocaine into the deltoid or vastus lateralis muscle.

and toxicity of local anesthetic agents is less following intranasal instillation and administration into the urethra and urinary bladder. Extremely low levels of lidocaine have been observed following the oral administration of this agent.[258, 259] These differences in absorption from various sites of topical application are due, in part, to the inherent variations in vascularity of the different anatomical sites and to the differences in pharmaceutical anesthetic preparations utilized

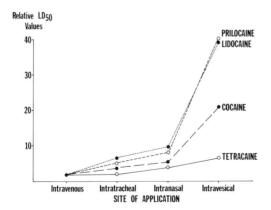

Fig. 5-4. Comparative toxicity of several local anesthetic agents as related to site of topical application.

for different forms of topical anesthesia. For example, the rapid absorption from the tracheobronchial tree is undoubtedly related not only to the vascularity of this area, but also to the use of anesthetic sprays which tend to disperse the anesthetic solution over a wide surface area and thus promote vascular absorption. On the other hand, local anesthetic agents are commonly employed in an ointment or gel form when applied to mucous membranes or instilled into the urethra. This formulation would tend to delay vascular absorption. The extremely low levels of lidocaine observed following oral administration may be due, in part, to a poor absorption from the gastrointestinal tract, but probably is more related to the rapid degradation of this agent as it is absorbed from the gastrointestinal tract and passes through the liver.[258, 259] For this reason, lidocaine, which is an effective antiarrhythmic drug when administered intravenously, is of little value orally in the treatment of cardiac arrhythmias.

Not only do local anesthetic agents vary in their absorption rates from various sites of topical application, but differences also exist between individual local anesthetic agents with regard to their relative absorption from specific sites. The toxicity of tetracaine following intratracheal instillation is similar to its intravenous toxicity, which suggests an extremely rapid rate of absorption following its administration into this particular site[124] (Fig. 5-4). Absorption from this particular site is apparently not so rapid for other agents such as lidocaine, prilocaine, and cocaine, since the acute toxicity following intratracheal administration of these agents is less than that observed after intravenous injection. Fatal reactions have been reported following the intratracheal administration of tetracaine for topical anesthesia, which probably reflects the rapid absorption of this particular drug from this site of administration.[260]

Dosage

The absorption and subsequent blood level of local anesthetic agents are related to the total dose of drug administered regardless of the site of administration (Fig. 5-5). For most agents, there is a linear relationship between the amount of drug administered and the resultant peak anesthetic blood level. For example, the mean venous blood level of lidocaine increased from approximately 1.5 μg/ml to 4 μg/ml as the total dose administered into the lumbar epidural space was increased from 200 to 600 mg. For certain local anesthetic agents, e.g., etidocaine, a nonlinear relationship exists between the total dose administered and the peak venous blood level (Fig. 5-6). This nonlinear-

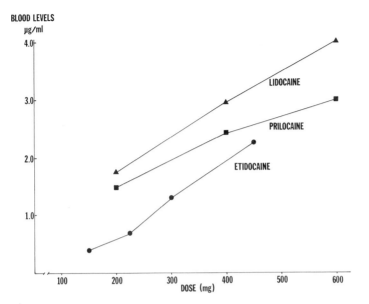

Fig. 5-5.   Peak venous plasma levels following epidural administration of varying doses of different anesthetic agents.

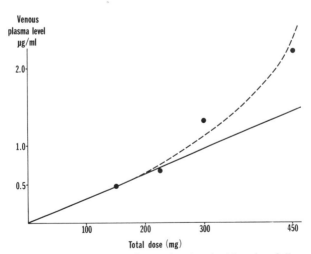

Fig. 5-6.   Peak venous plasma levels of etidocaine following epidural administration. Dashed line represents actual drug levels; solid line represents predicted drug levels.

ity has been observed following the lumbar epidural administration of etidocaine and may reflect the high lipid solubility of this agent, which results in a sequestration of the drug such that the rate of systemic absorption is less when relatively small dosages are used. However, when large doses are administered, lipid-binding sites may be saturated so that free drug is available for systemic absorption. [140, 200]

The peak anesthetic blood level achieved following regional anesthesia is a function of the total dose of drug administered and does not appear to be related to either the concentration or volume of the local anesthetic solution employed (Fig. 5-7). No significant differences in lidocaine, prilocaine, and etidocaine blood levels have been observed following the intercostal and epidural administration of these agents at varying volumes and concentrations, if the total dose was constant.[143,200] Moreover, lidocaine was administered intramuscularly in concentrations varying from 2% to 10% and no significant difference in peak venous blood levels was observed when the total dosage administered was unchanged[254, 255](Fig. 5-8). These results are consistent with the observations in Chapter 4 that anesthetic activity, in general, is related to the total dose of drug administered rather than to changes in concentration or volume of solution employed.

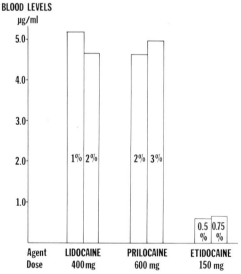

Fig. 5-7. Peak venous plasma levels following epidural administration of varying volumes and concentrations of several local anesthetic agents.

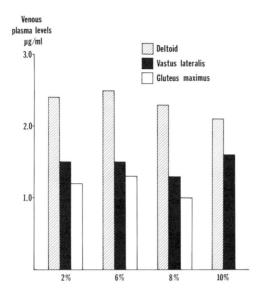

Fig. 5-8. Peak venous levels of lidocaine following intramuscular administration of varying concentrations and volumes of lidocaine (total dose = 300 mg).

Addition of Vasoconstrictor Agents

Many commercially prepared local anesthetic solutions contain a vasoconstrictor agent, usually epinephrine, in concentrations varying from 5 to 20 μg/ml. In addition, it is a common clinical practice to add epinephrine to plain solutions of local anesthetic drugs prior to their use for a variety of regional anesthetic procedures. The rationale for combining a vasoconstrictor agent with local anesthetic drugs is (a) to prolong the duration of action of certain local anesthetic agents by increasing neuronal uptake and (b) to decrease the rate of absorption from various sites of administration in order to reduce the potential systemic toxicity. Epinephrine in a concentration of 5 μg/ml (1:200,000) significantly reduces the peak blood levels of agents such as lidocaine and mepivacaine irrespective of the site of administration[143, 189] (Fig. 5-9). On the other hand, the peak blood levels of agents such as prilocaine, bupivacaine, and etidocaine appear to be minimally influenced by the addition of a vasoconstrictor substance[143, 200] (Fig. 5-9). The reasons for the apparent lack of absorption-retarding effect of epinephrine with these latter agents may differ depending on the specific drug. The lack of any difference between the peak blood levels of

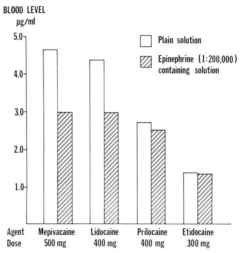

Fig. 5-9.   Effect of epinephrine on peak blood levels of various local anesthetic agents administered epidurally.

prilocaine following the lumbar epidural administration of either plain prilocaine or prilocaine with epinephrine may be attributable mainly to the extremely rapid rate of tissue redistribution of prilocaine.[261, 262] In the case of bupivacaine and etidocaine, the apparent lack of influence of epinephrine following lumbar epidural administration may be related, in part, to the high lipid solubility of these two agents, which results in a significant uptake by epidural adipose tissue and, also, to the greater vasodilating potential of bupivacaine and etidocaine, which may counteract the vasoconstricting effect of epinephrine.[22, 263]

The concentration of epinephrine that appears to be optimal in terms of reducing the rate of absorption of a local anesthetic agent such as lidocaine and mepivacaine from the lumbar epidural space is 5 μg/ml (1:200,000). The use of a 1:80,000 concentration of epinephrine was not associated with a significantly greater reduction in the peak blood level of lidocaine.[212] Other vasoconstrictor agents, such as phenylephrine and norepinephrine, have been employed in combination with local anesthetic agents. However, neither phenylephrine nor norepinephrine in concentrations of 1:20,000 appears to be as effective in reducing the rate of absorption of lidocaine and mepivacaine as epinephrine 1:200,000.[214, 264]

Pharmacological Characteristics of Local Anesthetic Agents

If all factors such as site of administration, dosage, and vasoconstrictor are maintained constant, the rate of absorption of local anesthetic agents will be determined by the chemical and pharmacological properties of the specific drug (Table 32). A comparison of agents of equivalent anesthetic potency reveals that lidocaine and mepivacaine show similar peak venous blood levels following lumbar epidural administration. Prilocaine blood levels are significantly lower than either lidocaine or mepivacaine, which may reflect the greater vasodilator activity of these latter agents (Table 32). The rapid rate of elimination of prilocaine also contributes to its lower blood levels as compared to lidocaine and mepivacaine.[24] Similarly, a comparison of the two more potent local anesthetic agents, bupivacaine and etidocaine, reveals that the peak blood level of etidocaine is significantly lower than that of bupivacaine following the lumbar epidural administration of equal doses of these two agents.[200] These differences in peak blood levels may be related, in part, to variations in the lipid solubility of these agents (Table 32). In addition, the rate of tissue redistribution of etidocaine is more rapid than that of bupivacaine, which produces lower blood levels.[265]

Unfortunately, no studies are available to compare the blood levels of the ester-type agents, e.g., procaine, chloroprocaine, and tetracaine following various forms of regional anesthesia. This is due, in part, to the rapid hydrolysis of these agents by plasma cholinesterase, which makes it difficult to measure the blood level of these substances and so determine the relative rates of absorption. How-

Table 32

INFLUENCE OF VASODILATOR ACTIVITY AND LIPID SOLUBILITY ON LOCAL ANESTHETIC ABSORPTION FROM EPIDURAL SPACE

Agent	Relative Vasodilator Activity	Approximate* Lipid Solubility	Maximum Blood Levels (Epidural Administration)	
			Dose (mg)	Conc. (µg/ml)
LIDOCAINE	1	2.9	300	1.4
PRILOCAINE	0.5	1.0	300	0.9
MEPIVACAINE	0.8	0.8	300	1.5
BUPIVACAINE	2.5	27.5	150	1.0
ETIDOCAINE	2.5	141	150	0.5

*n-Heptane/pH 7.4 buffer

ever, blood flow studies have shown that procaine,. chloroprocaine, and tetracaine cause vasodilation and, clinically, it is well known that epinephrine prolongs their anesthetic activity.[231,266] The only local anesthetic agent that consistently produces vasoconstriction is cocaine (Fig. 5-10). Direct blood flow measurements indicate that the initial effect of cocaine is one of vasodilation, followed by a prolonged state of vasoconstriction.[266] The mechanism of cocaine vaso-constriction is related to the inhibition of uptake of catecholamines into tissue-binding sites.[267] This inhibitory effect on catecholamine uptake, particularly norepinephrine, which results in less inactiva-tion of circulatory norepinephrine, is ultimately responsible for the prolonged state of vasoconstriction observed after administration of cocaine.

DISTRIBUTION OF LOCAL ANESTHETIC AGENTS

The blood level of local anesthetic agents following absorption from the site of injection is a function of both (a) rate of distribution from the vascular compartment to tissue compartments and (b) elimi-nation via metabolic and excretory pathways. Numerous reports are available in which the blood level of various local anesthetic agents has been measured. However, the values presented by different investigators may not be comparable due to variations in the defini-

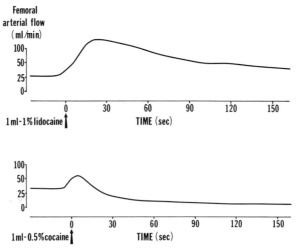

Fig. 5-10.   Effect of intraarterial injection of lidocaine and cocaine on femoral arterial blood flow in the dog.

tion of the phrase "blood concentration".[268] The level of a local anesthetic drug in blood may be expressed in terms of the base or hydrochloride salt of the specific agent under study. Often no indication is given in publications concerning which form of the drug is measured. Blood levels of lidocaine expressed as the HCl salt are approximately 10% to 15% higher than corresponding values expressed as the lidocaine base. Concentrations of local anesthetic agents are usually determined in either whole blood or plasma. These data are not necessarily interchangeable, since the degree of plasma protein-binding of various agents determines whether they are equally distributed between plasma and red blood cells. For example, prilocaine is poorly protein-bound and is distributed fairly evenly between plasma and red blood cells such that plasma and whole blood concentrations of this agent are quite similar. On the other hand, agents such as bupivacaine and etidocaine, which are highly protein-bound, show marked differences between plasma and whole blood concentrations (Table 33). Whole blood concentrations are lower than the plasma levels of agents which are highly protein-bound. A final distinction concerning local anesthetic blood levels must be made between arterial and venous blood concentration measurements. Most studies involve the determination of anesthetic drug levels in venous blood because of the ease of sampling. However, arterial blood concentrations of local anesthetic agents have been determined and are significantly higher than venous blood levels during the initial 60 minutes following drug injection.[268]

The disposition kinetics of local anesthetic agents can be calculated best following intravenous administration. The shape of the curve relating anesthetic concentration in blood to time, following IV injection, is similar for all agents (Fig. 5-11). Two or three disap-

Table 33

RELATIONSHIP BETWEEN PLASMA PROTEIN BINDING OF VARIOUS LOCAL ANESTHETIC AGENTS AND THEIR CONCENTRATION IN WHOLE BLOOD, PLASMA AND ERYTHROCYTES

Agent	% Plasma Protein Binding	Whole Blood Conc / Plasma Conc	Plasma Conc / RBC Conc
PRILOCAINE	55	1.0	0.88
LIDOCAINE	64	0.8	1.34- 2.1
MEPIVACAINE	77	0.7	2.6
ETIDOCAINE	94	0.5	7.5
BUPIVACAINE	95	0.5	7.8

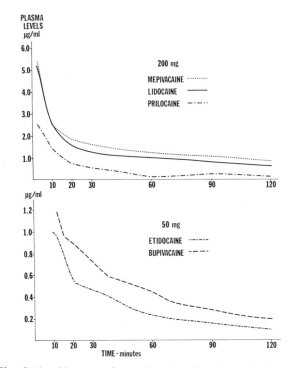

Fig. 5-11. Venous plasma levels of various local anesthetic agents following intravenous administration in man.

pearance phases have been described by various investigators.[259,265,268,269] The alpha phase represents the initial fast disappearance from blood into rapidly equilibrating tissues, i.e., tissue with
a high vascular perfusion. A secondary slower phase of disappearance (beta phase) is a function of distribution to slowly equilibrating
tissues and metabolism. This secondary disappearance phase has
been subdivided by some workers into a beta phase, i.e., distribution
to poorly perfused tissues and a gamma phase, i.e., elimination via
metabolic and excretory paths.

The rate of disappearance from blood usually is described in
terms of the time required for a 50% reduction in blood concentration
($T\frac{1}{2}$ or $T/2$). It is common to utilize the symbols $T/2\ \alpha$, $T/2\ \beta$, $T/2\ \gamma$
for the various disappearance phases. Local anesthetic agents show
different rates of disappearance from blood (Fig. 5-11). A comparison
of the three amide drugs of similar potency and duration of action,
i.e., lidocaine, mepivacaine, and prilocaine, reveals that the alpha and
beta half-lives of prilocaine are significantly shorter than those of

mepivacaine and lidocaine, which indicates a more rapid rate of redistribution from blood to tissues (Fig. 5-11).[262] The rate of tissue redistribution for lidocaine and mepivacaine is quite similar. The more potent, longer-acting amide anesthetic agents, i.e., bupivacaine and etidocaine, possess higher $T/2 \, \alpha$ and $T/2 \, \beta$ values than the less potent agents of this class.[265,268] However, etidocaine possesses shorter alpha and beta half-lives than bupivacaine, which implies a more rapid rate of tissue redistribution (Fig. 5-11).[265,268] The rate of tissue redistribution appears related, in part, to the protein-binding and lipid solubility characteristics of the various agents. In general, compounds that are poorly protein-bound, e.g., prilocaine, and highly lipid soluble, e.g., etidocaine, distribute themselves more rapidly between blood and tissues.

The volume of distribution (V_D) is a calculated kinetic parameter which has been used to evaluate the distributive properties of drugs. V_D does not represent a true physiological space, but is indicative of the apparent distribution of a drug in the body with respect to the dose administered and the concentration in blood. The relative volume of distribution provides information concerning the differential uptake and accumulation of local anesthetic agents by various body tissues. For example, highly lipid-soluble drugs tend to accumulate in adipose tissue and so appear to have a large volume of distribution. Tucker and Mather have calculated the volume of distribution of various amide local anesthetic agents under steady state conditions, which they believe characterizes more accurately the relative distribution of the different drugs (Fig. 5-12).[268]

Local anesthetic agents are distributed throughout all body tissues, but the relative concentration in different tissues varies[24, 27, 270-272] (Fig. 5-13). In general, the more highly perfused organs such as the lung and kidney show higher local anesthetic concentrations than less well-perfused organs (Fig. 5-13). Skeletal muscle contains the highest percentage of the total injected dose of a local anesthetic agent, although the concentration of local anesthetic agent per gram of muscle tissue is not large. However, skeletal muscle is the largest mass of tissue in the body and serves as the greatest reservoir for local anesthetic agents.

Differences exist between the tissue levels of various local anesthetic agents. For example, Sung and Truant compared the distribution of procaine and lidocaine in rats and observed higher levels of lidocaine in fat tissue and in liver.[27] A comparative study of prilocaine and lidocaine in rats revealed the presence of significantly higher concentrations of prilocaine in lung tissue.[24] Mepivacaine

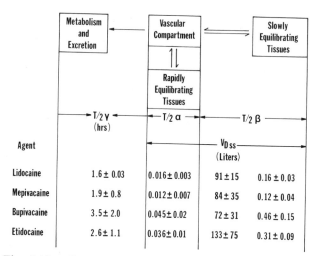

Fig. 5-12. Comparative pharmacokinetic properties of various local anesthetic agents calculated according to a three-compartment model.

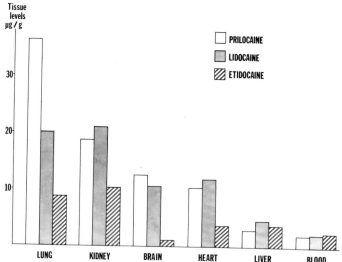

Fig. 5-13. Peak tissue levels of prilocaine, lidocaine, and etidocaine in guinea pigs following subcutaneous administration.

showed a distribution pattern similar to that of lidocaine, with a rapid accumulation in liver, kidney, salivary glands, and brain.[273] A comparison of the tissue levels of etidocaine and bupivacaine in guinea pigs demonstrated the previously mentioned accumulation of etidocaine in adipose tissue (Table 34).

Selective tissue distribution studies have been conducted in man. As indicated previously, the comparative plasma/erythrocyte (P/E) distribution of various local anesthetic agents has been determined and correlated directly with the relative protein-binding of the specific drugs (Table 33).[21,261] Prilocaine shows the lowest degree of plasma-protein-binding and the lowest P/E ratio, whereas bupivacaine is bound to the greatest degree to plasma proteins and has the highest P/E ratio.

The degree of uptake of local anesthetic agents by skeletal muscle also has been approximated in man by the simultaneous measurement of anesthetic blood levels in brachial artery and antecubital vein. The peripheral venous/arterial blood concentration ratio for lidocaine was reported to be 0.73 ± 0.003 compared to a value of 0.47 ± 0.003 for prilocaine, which is indicative of the more rapid tissue redistribution of prilocaine.[261] Similar studies with bupivacaine and etidocaine reveal 20% to 40% higher levels of these agents in arterial samples than in simultaneously drawn venous samples.[209, 268] These studies in man are consistent with the distribution studies in animals, which indicate a rapid tissue uptake for all local anesthetic agents, but differences in the rate and degree of tissue redistribution between specific local anesthetic drugs as a function of their intrinsic physicochemical properties.

The rate of tissue uptake of local anesthetic agents will be influenced by the physiological status of the subject.[273] The rate of

Table 34

TISSUE (μg/ g)/ BLOOD (μg /ml) RATIOS OF ETIDOCAINE
AND BUPIVACAINE IN THE GUINEA PIG

TISSUE	ETIDOCAINE	BUPIVACAINE
BRAIN	1.3	3.5
HEART	1.8	3.9
FAT	7.8	4.4
MUSCLE	0.8	1.3

lidocaine disappearance from blood is significantly prolonged in patients with a decreased vascular perfusion of tissues secondary to impaired myocardial contractility.[274] The arteriovenous difference of lidocaine and etidocaine was considerably greater in human volunteers undergoing epidural blockade compared to surgical patients during the initial 60 minutes following administration into the lumbar epidural space. These data suggest a more rapid rate of tissue uptake by the healthy volunteers.[268]

A special category of local anesthetic distribution involves placental transmission and uptake by fetal tissue. Considerable information has been obtained in recent years concerning the placental transmission of local anesthetic agents.[275-286] In general, local anesthetic drugs appear to cross the placenta by passive diffusion. However, the rate and degree of diffusion vary considerably between specific agents and appear to be inversely correlated with the degree of plasma-protein-binding (Table 35).[287] Prilocaine shows the highest umbilical vein/maternal blood (UV/M) ratio (1.00–1.08) and lowest plasma-protein-binding capacity (55%).[279, 281] On the other hand, the UV/M ratio of bupivacaine and etidocaine is 0.14–0.44 and these agents are approximately 95% protein-bound.[282, 285, 286] Lidocaine and mepivacaine occupy an intermediate position both in terms of placental transmission (UV/M ratio of 0.52–0.71) and protein-binding (64–77%).[275-278,280,283,284]

The placental transmission of local anesthetic agents does not appear to be influenced by the route of administration. For example, the UV/M ratio of lidocaine was similar following paracervical, lumbar epidural, and IV administration.[277, 278] The peak venous plasma level of local anesthetic agents in maternal blood also does not affect placental transfer. The UV/M ratio of mepivacaine in two separate investigations were similar (0.69 and 0.71), whereas the maternal blood levels showed a twofold difference (2.9 and 6.9 μg/ml).[275, 280]

Table 35

RELATIONSHIP BETWEEN PLASMA PROTEIN BINDING CAPACITY AND UMBILICAL VEIN/
MATERNAL BLOOD (UV/M) RATIO OF VARIOUS LOCAL ANESTHETIC AGENTS

Agent	Protein Binding Capacity %	Maternal Arterial or Venous Blood Levels(μg/ml)	Umbilical Vein Levels(μg/ml)	UV/M Ratio
PRILOCAINE	55	1.03-1.5	1.07-1.5	1.0-1.18
LIDOCAINE	64	1.23-3.5	0.8-1.8	0.52-0.69
MEPIVACAINE	77	2.91-6.9	1.9-4.9	0.69-0.71
BUPIVACAINE	95	0.26	0.08-0.11	0.31-0.44
ETIDOCAINE	94	0.25-1.3	0.07-0.45	0.14-0.35

The comparative maternal and fetal tissue distribution of local anesthetic drugs have been investigated by Finster and co-workers in guinea pigs.[288, 289] Although the distribution of lidocaine in maternal and fetal tissues was generally similar, certain differences did exist (Table 36). For example, significantly higher levels of lidocaine were found in fetal liver than in adult liver. This may be indicative of poorly developed enzyme systems in the fetus such that amide-type local anesthetic drugs may not be metabolized as rapidly in fetal liver as in adult liver. Studies comparing etidocaine and lidocaine revealed a greater uptake by fetal brain of etidocaine than of lidocaine.[289] Etidocaine tends to accumulate in peripheral fat in adults; the lack of peripheral fat depots in the fetus could result in the uptake of this agent by other lipid organs such as brain. In summary, the placental transmission of local anesthetic agents is influenced mainly by the degree of maternal plasma-protein-binding of the various agents and the rate of fetal tissue uptake.[290] Fetal plasma-binding of local anesthetic agents is approximately 50% less than binding in maternal plasma, so that more unbound drug is present in the fetus.[291] Those drugs that demonstrate the highest degree of protein-binding also tend to be more lipid soluble, such that the rate of tissue uptake of the unbound drug is enhanced. Thus, the maternal/fetal anesthetic blood concentrations may differ markedly between agents, but the total amount of drug transferred across the placenta may be similar for agents of high and lower protein-binding capacity. The clinical significance of these findings is not certain. It was originally postulated that agents which possess a high protein-binding capacity should be potentially less toxic for the fetus.[22] However, if the rate of fetal tissue uptake is greater for drugs of high protein-binding and high lipid solubility, then the potential fetal toxicity would be similar for all of the local anesthetic compounds.

Table 36

COMPARATIVE GUINEA PIG MATERNAL AND FETAL
TISSUE LEVELS OF LIDOCAINE

TISSUE	PEAK MATERNAL LEVEL	PEAK FETAL LEVEL
BLOOD (μg/ml)	7.6	3.6
MYOCARDIUM (μg/g)	17.2	8.9
BRAIN	31.9	9.7
KIDNEY	42.3	5.8
LIVER	7.8	22.9

METABOLISM

The metabolism of local anesthetic agents is related to their basic chemical structure. As indicated previously, the clinically useful compounds can be separated into two general classes: agents containing an ester linkage (e.g., procaine and tetracaine) and agents containing an amide linkage (e.g., lidocaine and mepivacaine).

Ester Compounds

The ester or procaine class of local anesthetic drugs are hydrolyzed in plasma by the enzyme, pseudocholinesterase.[26] The rate of hydrolysis may vary markedly between agents in this chemical class.[23] Chloroprocaine shows the most rapid rate of hydrolysis (4.7 μmoles/ml/hour), while a rate of 1.1 μmoles/ml/hour was observed for procaine and 0.3 μmoles/ml hour for tetracaine[23] (Table 3). The anesthetic quality and potential toxicity of ester-type agents appear to bear an inverse correlation to the rate of hydrolysis. Thus, tetracaine, which exerts the longest duration of anesthesia and is the most toxic of the ester-type local anesthetic agents, undergoes the slowest rate of hydrolysis, whereas 2-chloroprocaine, which possesses the shortest duration of anesthetic action and is the least toxic agent, is the most rapidly hydrolyzed. Procaine occupies an intermediate position, both in terms of anesthetic duration, systemic toxicity, and rate of hydrolysis. This type of metabolic pathway has specific clinical relevance, since subjects with atypical forms of pseudocholinesterase may be incapable of hydrolyzing agents of the procaine-type, which could result in a prolongation of systemic toxic effects.[292]

Some of the metabolites formed by the hydrolysis of the various ester-type agents have been identified.[26] For example, procaine undergoes cleavage at the ester linkage to form para-aminobenzoic acid and diethylamino ethanol. Para-aminobenzoic acid then is excreted unchanged in the urine, whereas diethylamino ethanol may undergo further metabolism. The type of metabolites formed from the parent local anesthetic compounds also is of clinical significance. The allergic phenomena which occur more frequently with the use of the ester-type local anesthetic agents are not related to the parent compounds, such as procaine and tetracaine, but are attributable to the formation of para-aminobenzoic acid, the primary metabolite formed from the hydrolysis of procaine, chloroprocaine, and tetracaine.

Amide Compounds

The metabolism of the amide-type anesthetic agents is more complex than that of the ester agents. A number of studies performed in animals and man have revealed that the liver is the prime site of metabolism for these amide-type drugs. Sung and Truant compared the rate of metabolism of lidocaine incubated with various rat tissue slices and found the liver to be the most active organ for metabolizing this agent.[27] Similar in vitro studies with mepivacaine have shown that this agent is readily metabolized by rat liver slices incubated under aerobic conditions.[28] Prilocaine appears to differ somewhat from lidocaine and mepivacaine. Although this agent is readily metabolized by rat liver slices, some degradation also occurs when prilocaine is incubated with kidney slices.[293] Isolated liver perfusion studies with bupivacaine and etidocaine have revealed that these compounds also undergo hepatic degradation.[294]

In vivo studies have confirmed the in vitro tissue slice data, indicating that the liver is the prime site of metabolism for local anesthetic agents of the amide-type. Studies in rats have shown that hepatectomy results in substantially higher tissue levels of lidocaine and an increase in the anesthetic activity and duration of toxic symptoms produced by this agent.[27] The rate of disappearance of lidocaine from blood was also found to decrease in hepatectomized dogs and in patients whose livers had been removed during the course of liver transplantation.[295]

Differences exist between the amide-type local anesthetic agents with regard to their relative rates of metabolism (Table 37).[24, 28, 294] Prilocaine has been shown to undergo the most rapid rate of degradation in liver slices, whereas the rate of metabolism of lidocaine, mepivacaine, bupivacaine, and etidocaine appear to be similar. The degradation of the amide-type local anesthetic agents is influenced by the hepatic status of the individual subject. Simultaneous measurements of arterial and hepatic venous levels of lidocaine and estimations of hepatic blood flow have shown that approximately 70% of injected lidocaine is metabolized in subjects with normal liver function.[296] In patients in whom liver blood flow is abnormally low, or in whom liver function is poor or nonexistent, the breakdown of the amide-type of local anesthetic agent is markedly decreased, resulting in significantly higher blood levels which, in turn, may potentially lead to greater toxicity of this class of drugs.[295] Indeed, systemic reactions to lidocaine have been reported in patients with severe hepatic disease.[297]

Table 37

COMPARATIVE RATES OF METABOLISM AND METABOLITES OF VARIOUS AMIDE LOCAL ANESTHETIC AGENTS

Agent	Metabolic rate*	Chemical nomenclature	Metabolic products
PRILOCAINE	> 90	2-propylamino-o-propionotoluidide	o-toluidine, L-N-n-propylamine
LIDOCAINE	62	Diethylaminoacet-2,6-xylidide	monoethylglycinexylidide, 3-hydroxy-lidocaine, 3-hydroxy- monoethylglycinexylidide, 2,6 xylidine, glycinexylidide, 4-hydroxy-2,6-dimethylaniline, 2-amino-3-methylbenzoic acid
MEPIVACAINE	55	1-N-methylpipecolic acid 2,6-dimethylanalide	2,6-pipecoloxylidide-3-hydroxy-1-methyl, 2,6-pipecoloxylidine, 2,6-pipecoloxylidide 4-hydroxy-1-methyl
BUPIVACAINE	54	1-butyl-2,6-pipecoloxylidide	2,6-pipecoloxylidine
ETIDOCAINE	67	2-(N-ethylpropylamino)-2,6-butyroxylidide	2,6 xylidine, 2-ethylamino-2,6-butyroxylidide, 2-propylamino-2,6-butyroxylidide, 2-amino-butyroxylidide

*Percent metabolites appearing following 10-30 minutes of incubation or perfusion of guinea pig or rat liver slices

Although many of the primary metabolites of the various amide agents have been identified (Table 36),[298] the complete spectrum of metabolic products derived from the compounds in this class has not been elucidated. The metabolism of lidocaine has been studied most extensively (Fig. 5-14). Hollunger originally proposed a metabolic pathway for the degradation of lidocaine in rat and rabbit liver.[299] The initial step involved the oxidative deethylation of lidocaine to monoethylglycinexylidide and acetaldehyde. Monoethylglycinexylidide subsequently was hydrolyzed to xylidine and monoethylglycine. Xylidine itself underwent further oxidation to some unknown product. Keenaghan and Boyes summarized the information available concerning the metabolism of lidocaine in various animals species and demonstrated considerable species variability.[300] Significant amounts of monoethylglycinexylidide and xylidine were recovered from guinea pig urine. Rats formed large quantities of the meta-hydroxy derivative of both lidocaine and monoethylglycinexylidide. These phenolic derivatives appear to a limited extent in dogs and man. The conjugates of these two metabolites were extensively recycled in the bile of rats. However, these metabolites were essentially lacking in man, which suggests that biliary recycling is not a significant pathway for lidocaine elimination in man. Hydroxyxylidine was the major metabolic product of lidocaine found in dog and human urine. The dog and human were most similar in terms of lidocaine metabolism, whereas the rat and man appeared quite dissimilar. A number of

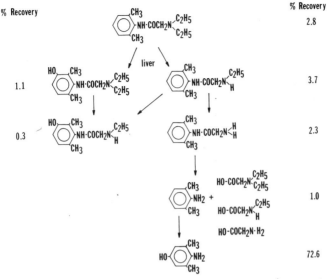

Fig. 5-14. Suggested metabolism of lidocaine in man and percent recovery of various metabolites in human urine.

minor metabolites of lidocaine have been described by various investigators.[301, 302] However, some confusion has existed concerning whether these substances are actually formed from the degradation of lidocaine or represent artifacts of the experimental analytical system.[303, 304]

The metabolism of mepivacaine has been studied in liver slice preparations from mice and rats, and n-demethylation appears to be the initial step in the degradation of this agent in these species.[28] Hydroxylation of mepivacaine also occurs in rats and man, and as observed with lidocaine, approximately 60% of the dose of mepivacaine administered to rats is excreted as an aromatic hydroxy derivative.[305]

In man, conjugates of these hydroxy metabolites of mepivacaine account for 25% to 40% of the administered dose of mepivacaine.[305, 306] In addition, three neutral metabolites of mepivacaine have been identified in human urine,[307] but approximately 50% of administered mepivacaine remains unidentified. Meffin, Long, and Thomas have also studied the metabolism of mepivacaine in human neonates and suggest that the newborn is not capable of aromatic hydroxylation of mepivacaine.[308]

The metabolism of prilocaine differs significantly from that of lidocaine and mepivacaine, due apparently to the lack of one methyl group on the aromatic portion of the molecule (Table 1). o-toluidine and L-N-n-propylamine have been identified as metabolites of prilocaine.[293] These substances also may undergo further degradation.

Detailed metabolic data are not available on the newer amide-type of local anesthetic agents, i.e., bupivacaine and etidocaine. Preliminary studies by Reynolds in which the metabolism of bupivacaine and mepivacaine was compared in human volunteers revealed that approximately 5% of the dose of bupivacaine administered was recovered in urine as the N-dealkylated metabolite, pipecolylxylidine.[309] Goehl and associates studied the metabolism of bupivacaine in rats and monkeys and observed that the rat excretes substantial quantities of bupivacaine as an aromatic hydroxy metabolite, whereas the monkey excretes over 50% of the dose as the hydrolysis product, pipecolic acid.[310]

Preliminary data on the metabolism of etidocaine, which is structurally similar to lidocaine, have shown that only 1.1% of the administered dose of etidocaine was recovered in guinea pig urine as the secondary amine metabolite, whereas 14.9% of lidocaine was identified as the secondary amine metabolite.[298] The excretion of 2,6-xylidine in guinea pigs was also considerably lower following etidocaine administration (2.2%) than following lidocaine administration (16.2%). The presence of the branched alkyl chain in etidocaine probably results in metabolic products that are markedly different than those of lidocaine.

The products formed from the degradation of the amide-type local anesthetic agents may have clinically significant implications. Under normal physiological conditions, these metabolites exert relatively insignificant pharmacological or toxicological effects. In certain situations, however, such as renal or cardiac failure, or during prolonged periods of administration, these metabolites might accumulate and exert significant clinical effects. For example, certain metabolites of lidocaine have been shown to possess antiarrhythmic and toxicological properties similar to, but less potent than, that of the parent compound lidocaine.[311] Other lidocaine metabolites may accumulate in the plasma of patients following prolonged intravenous therapy with lidocaine for control of cardiac arrhythmias and may produce systemic toxic effects that are additive to the inherent toxicity of the parent compound, lidocaine.[312] The prime example of a metabolite being responsible for the toxicity of a local anesthetic agent is the methemoglobinemia that occurs in patients treated with large doses of prilocaine.[25] Prilocaine, itself, is not capable of producing methemoglobin. However, o-toluidine, which is one of the main metabolites of prilocaine, can induce the formation of methemoglobin in vitro and is believed responsible for the methemoglobinemia observed in man.

EXCRETION

The kidney is the main excretory organ for local anesthetic agents and their metabolites. Among the ester class of local anesthetic drugs, procaine is hydrolyzed almost completely in plasma and less than 2% of unchanged drug is excreted by the kidney.[26] Approximately 90% of para-aminobenzoic acid, the primary metabolite of procaine, is found unchanged in the urine, whereas only one-third of diethylaminoethanol, the other metabolite, is excreted unchanged. Similarly, only small amounts of unchanged chloroprocaine and tetracaine are found in urine.

Only small amounts of the amide-type local anesthetic agents are excreted unchanged via the kidneys. Less than 10% of intravenously administered lidocaine was found in the urine of human volunteers.[300, 313] Approximately 80% of administered lidocaine could be recovered in human urine in the form of various metabolites.[300] From 1% to 16% of administered mepivacaine appears as unchanged drug in human urine, whereas 25% to 40% is excreted as degradation products.[305,306,309] Only 16% of unchanged bupivacaine has been recovered from human urine.[309] Cocaine is the only local anesthetic agent of either the ester or amide-type that is excreted mainly in an unchanged form in kidney.[245]

A study of the comparative renal clearance of prilocaine and lidocaine in man by Eriksson and Granberg indicated a substantially higher clearance value for prilocaine, which they believed to be related to the lower protein binding of prilocaine.[314] The renal clearance of both prilocaine and lidocaine was found to be inversely proportional to the pH of urine, which suggests that the urinary excretion of these agents occurred by nonionic diffusion. This finding may have practical clinical implications, since urinary acidification may provide a means of increasing the excretion of local anesthetic agents in patients in whom toxic symptoms develop.

Biliary excretion appears to play a role in the disposition of local anesthetic agents in certain animal species. Lidocaine, mepivacaine, and tetracaine or their metabolites have been isolated from bile.[1, 28, 300, 315] In rodents, unchanged tetracaine is excreted by way of the common bile duct into the gastrointestinal tract and then completely reabsorbed into blood, where hydrolysis occurs. The metabolites are ultimately excreted via the kidneys. On the other hand, lidocaine and mepivacaine undergo hepatic degradation initially, following which some of the metabolites are excreted by way of the common bile duct into the gastrointestinal tract. The metabolites are then completely reabsorbed and ultimately appear in urine. The biliary excretion and recycling of lidocaine appear to be important in eliminating this agent in rats, but probably are not significant in either dog or man.[298]

SUMMARY

1. The physiological disposition of local anesthetic agents can be summarized as follows (Fig. 5-15): (1) complete absorption from the site of injection into the central vascular compartment; (2) redistribution throughout total body water according to a 2- or 3-compartment pharmacokinetic model, with the rate of tissue redistribution varying as a function of such physicochemical properties as protein-binding capacity and lipid solubility; (3) metabolism of the ester-type agents in blood by the enzyme, pseudocholinesterase, with amide agents undergoing degradation primarily in the liver; (4) biliary recycling of the parent compound itself or metabolites in some animal species; (5) excretion of the remaining unchanged drug and metabolites via the kidney into the urine.

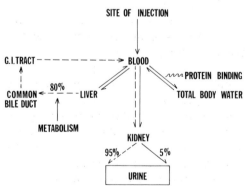

Fig. 5-15. Physiological disposition of local anesthetic agents.

2. The metabolism and elimination of local anesthetic agents can be significantly influenced by the clinical status of the patient which, in turn, may effect the potential toxicity of this class of compounds. For example, the average half-life of lidocaine in blood of approximately 90 minutes in normal subjects is markedly prolonged in patients with significant degree of cardiac failure. The rate of hydrolysis of the ester agents is decreased in patients with atypical forms of the enzyme, pseudocholinesterase, while hepatic dysfunction will result in an accumulation of the amide-type local anesthetic agents. The kidney is the prime excretory organ for both unchanged drug and the metabolites of local anesthetic agents. A significant impairment of renal function may result in increased blood levels of the parent compound or its metabolites which may cause adverse systemic effects.

6

General Pharmacological and Toxicological Aspects of Local Anesthetic Agents

Local anesthetic agents are usually applied to the specific area of the body where they exert their primary pharmacological action of conduction blockade. However, as discussed in Chapter 5, local anesthetic drugs are absorbed systemically and can affect organs other than peripheral nerves. Since these drugs may act on any excitable membranes, the cardiovascular and central nervous systems are particularly susceptible to the action of local anesthetic agents.

CENTRAL NERVOUS SYSTEM EFFECTS

Local anesthetic agents readily cross the blood-brain barrier to cause alterations in the central nervous system (CNS).

Behavioral and EEG Alterations

In general, a consistent sequence of events is observed following a progressive increase in the dose and subsequent blood level of a local anesthetic agent. At nontoxic levels, minimal CNS changes occur; the initial signs of CNS toxicity are usually excitatory in nature. Various symptoms have been described by human volunteers receiving intravenous local anesthetic drugs.[265, 316–318] Numbness of the tongue and circumoral tissues is the earliest subjective symptom and probably does not reflect a CNS effect, but rather a high local tissue concentration of drug in this highly vascular area. A generalized feeling of lightheadedness and dizziness is the first indication of CNS alterations, followed by visual and auditory disturbances, such as difficulty in focusing and tinnitus. Drowsiness, disorientation, and temporary unconsciousness have also been reported. Objective signs of early CNS toxicity consist of slurred speech, shivering, muscular twitching and tremors in muscles of the face and distal parts of the extremities. Electroencephalographic recordings do not correlate well with these early subjective and objective signs and symptoms. The appearance of slow waves and an increased amount of delta-theta activity and a decrease in alpha activity have been observed in the EEG of some subjects.[228, 316]

Electroencephalographic studies in animals have revealed that the amygdala shows the most consistent changes in activity following administration of local anesthetic agents. Subconvulsive doses of lidocaine are usually associated with an electrical pattern described as rhythmic spindling.[319] Slow high-voltage cortical activity appears after the onset of changes in the amygdala. As the dose and subsequent blood level of a local anesthetic agent are increased, these initial CNS signs and symptoms progress into a generalized convulsive state of a tonic-clonic nature. This overt convulsive activity is correlated with amygdaloid spike-spindle complexes, spiking, and finally ictal episodes of a generalized nature.[319] Following this period of CNS excitation, a further increase in the amount of local anesthetic drug administered results in cessation of seizure activity and a flattening of the brain-wave pattern, consistent with generalized CNS depression. Respiratory depression and ultimately respiratory arrest are the overt manifestations of this CNS depressive state.

Since local anesthetic agents generally exert a depressant effect on excitable membranes, the cause of the initial central nervous system excitation has been a subject of considerable interest. The mechanism of the initial CNS excitation and subsequent depression is explained by the stabilizing effect of local anesthetic agents on cell membranes. Convulsive doses of lidocaine produce initially a blockade of inhibitory pathways in the cerebral cortex.[319-323] The specific site of action involves either inhibitory cortical synapses[320, 321] or inhibitory cortical neurons.[323] This inhibition of inhibitory pathways allows facilitory neurons to function unopposed, leading to an increase in excitation of the CNS, ultimately manifested in convulsive activity. Further increases in dose produce a depression of both inhibitory and facilitory pathways, which results in a generalized state of CNS depression.[319]

Factors Influencing the CNS Effects of Local Anesthetic Agents

The convulsive action of local anesthetic agents is a function of the specific drug employed, the acid-base status of the patient, and the concomitant use of other CNS active agents.

LOCAL ANESTHETIC AGENT

Acute intravenous toxicity studies in animals[324-328] and human intravenous tolerance studies[23,316-318] have revealed that the dose of a local anesthetic agent required to produce preconvulsive signs and symptoms in man and frank convulsions in animals is directly related to the intrinsic anesthetic potency of the compound. For example, procaine which shows the lowest intrinsic anesthetic potency of the clinically useful local anesthetic agents, possesses the highest convulsive ED_{50} value, i.e., the dose which will produce convulsions in 50% of animals following a rapid IV injection. On the other hand, bupivacaine, which is intrinsically a very potent compound, exhibits a very low convulsive ED_{50} value (Fig. 6-1).[327] Lidocaine, mepivacaine, and prilocaine are intermediate both with respect to anesthetic potency and convulsive activity.[326]

The convulsive threshold of local anesthetic agents also has been defined in terms of the anesthetic blood level associated with the onset of seizure activity[325,326,328] and again is directly related to intrinsic anesthetic potency. For example, bupivacaine produces convulsions in

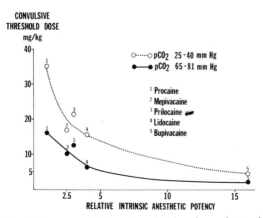

Fig. 6-1. The convulsive threshold of various local anesthetic agents as related to their intrinsic anesthetic potency and arterial pCO_2.

monkeys at a blood level of 5.5 μg/ml, whereas lidocaine-induced convulsions occur at a blood level of 26 μg/ml (Table 38).[326] A precise correlation has not been observed between venous blood levels of local anesthetic agents and CNS alterations in man.[316,318] Scott has demonstrated that the administration of etidocaine to the same subject resulted in symptoms of CNS toxicity at a venous plasma level of 2.6 μg/ml on one occasion and no signs of CNS toxicity at a venous plasma level of 3.7 μg/ml on a second occasion.[318] Possibly, arterial blood levels may serve as a more precise predictor of CNS toxicity than venous anesthetic levels. Moreover, the rate of IV administration is also an important determinant of the toxic threshold of a particular agent.[319]

Although all local anesthetic agents can induce convulsions, the preconvulsive alterations in CNS activity may vary depending on the specific local anesthetic drug administered. Subconvulsive doses of lidocaine and procaine are often associated with sedative-like symptoms of drowsiness and temporary loss of consciousness.[316,317] This type of behavioral change has not been described for other local anesthetic agents. EEG recordings in monkeys treated with lidocaine have also shown a characteristic preconvulsive pattern of diffuse slowing and irregular appearance of large spikes and slow waves leading directly into general seizure activity (Fig. 6-2).[325,328] Other local anesthetic agents such as mepivacaine, bupivacaine, and etidocaine do not consistently produce distinctive preconvulsive EEG changes. Usually a generalized seizure pattern, at the time of overt convulsions, is the only EEG alteration observed[325,326,328] (Fig. 6-2).

Table 38

THRESHOLD FOR PRODUCTION OF CNS TOXICITY BY VARIOUS LOCAL ANESTHETIC AGENTS

Agent	Convulsive threshold Monkey*		Convulsive threshold Cat**	Threshold-CNS symptoms Man		
	Dose-mg/Kg	Arterial blood level-μg/ml	Dose mg/Kg	Dose mg/Kg 1	2	3
PROCAINE	—	—	50	18−55	19.2	—
CHLOROPROCAINE	—	—	—	—	22.8	—
LIDOCAINE	14−22	18−26	22	6−9	6.4	>4
MEPIVACAINE	18	22	21	—	9.8	—
PRILOCAINE	18	20	35	—	—	>6
BUPIVACAINE	4.3	4.5−5.5	5.8	—	—	1.6
ETIDOCAINE	5.4	4.3	—	—	—	3.4
TETRACAINE	—	—	—	—	2.5	—

* data from Munson (326,328)   ** data from Englesson (334)
1 "   " Usubiaga (317)
2 "   " Foldes (23)
3 "   " Scott (318)

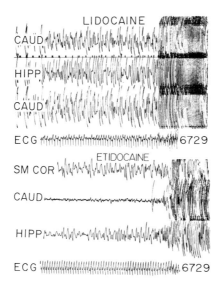

Fig. 6-2. EEG changes in one monkey (6729) following the IV administration of a convulsive dose of lidocaine and of etidocaine. Preconvulsive EEG changes are noted during the lidocaine infusion, but not during etidocaine administration. (Courtesy of Dr. E. Munson.)

ACID-BASE STATUS

The relationship of pH and pCO_2 to the convulsive threshold of various local anesthetic agents has been studied by several investigators.[319,327,329] In general, the convulsive threshold is inversely related to the arterial pCO_2 level. An increase in pCO_2 is associated with a reduction in the dosage and blood level of local anesthetic agent required to induce seizures, whereas a decrease in pCO_2 requires that a greater amount of local analgesic drug be administered in order to produce convulsive activity. For example, Englesson has reported that the convulsive threshold dose of procaine in cats was decreased from approximately 35 mg/kg to 15 mg/kg when the pCO_2 was elevated from 25–40 torr to 65–81 torr (Fig. 6-1).[327] Similar changes in convulsive threshold were observed with mepivacaine, prilocaine, lidocaine, and bupivacaine.

A decrease in arterial pH also will decrease the convulsive threshold of local anesthetic agents.[327] A study of the interrelationship between pCO_2, pH, and local anesthetic activity has shown that respiratory acidosis always decreases the convulsive threshold of local anesthetic agents, but the degree of threshold alteration is dependent on the underlying metabolic condition.[327] A high pCO_2, associated with a decrease in arterial pH due to metabolic acidosis, will cause a greater decrease in convulsive threshold than the same pCO_2 level which is achieved in the presence of a normal or elevated arterial pH, i.e., metabolic alkalosis.

Several mechanisms have been postulated to explain the inverse relation between arterial CO_2 tension and local anesthetic convulsive threshold.[329] An elevated pCO_2 may enhance cerebral blood flow so that more anesthetic agent is delivered to the brain or may exert an excitatory CNS effect which is additive to or potentiates the convulsive action of local anesthetic drugs. A high pCO_2 also may produce a fall in intracellular pH which, in turn, will cause an increase in the intraneuronal level of the active cationic form of the local anesthetic agent.

The seizures induced by local anesthetic drugs may be prolonged by certain feedback mechanisms related to changes produced by the convulsive activity. A progressive metabolic acidosis occurs during the period of generalized seizures, which tends to prolong the hyperexcitable CNS state as the local anesthetic blood level declines.[330] In addition, an increase in cerebral metabolism and cerebral blood flow has been reported during local anesthetic-induced convulsions. Such increases would deliver more drug to the brain, which would prolong the period of seizure activity.[331]

CONCOMITANT USE OF OTHER
CNS ACTIVE AGENTS

The convulsive threshold of local anesthetic agents can be increased by the prior or concomitant administration of CNS depressant drugs such as diazepam, barbiturates, and general anesthesia.[332-335] Premedication with 0.25 mg/kg of diazepam intramuscularly produced a 100% increase in the convulsive ED_{50} of lidocaine in cats,[332] whereas ventilation with 70% nitrous oxide caused a 50% increase in the convulsive ED_{50} of lidocaine. No additive protective effect was observed when 70% inspired N_2O and diazepam were employed together prior to the administration of a convulsive dose of lidocaine.[334] An increase in the convulsive threshold of lidocaine persisted for at least 5 hours following pretreatment of cats with diazepam.[335]

Studies involving the prophylactive use of barbiturates to alter the convulsive threshold of local anesthetic agents have yielded conflicting results. No difference in seizure activity has been reported by some workers following the administration of local analgesic agents to rats and man pretreated with thiopental.[317,336] Other investigators have demonstrated a prophylactic anticonvulsant action of pentobarbital.[337,338] A comparison of 0.25 mg/kg diazepam and 10 mg/kg pentobarbital by de Jong and Heavner revealed a similar protection against lidocaine-induced seizures in cats. However, the pentobarbital-lidocaine-treated animals exhibited a greater degree of CNS and cardiorespiratory depression than did the diazepam-lidocaine-treated group.[338]

Although some discrepancies may exist concerning the relative merits of diazepam and barbiturates in the prevention of local anesthetic-induced convulsions, both types of agents are effective in terminating seizure activity produced by local anesthetic drugs. Intravenous thiopental (4 mg/kg) and diazepam (0.1 mg/kg) have been demonstrated to rapidly stop both EEG and muscle seizures in man and monkeys.[317,339]

Neuromuscular blocking agents also have been employed to prevent or reverse local anesthetic-induced convulsions. Munson and Wagman have demonstrated that gallamine can increase the lidocaine threshold for electrical seizure activity in monkeys from 26 μg/ml to 36 μg/ml.[340] Usubiaga and co-workers reported that succinylcholine terminated muscle seizure activity in man, but did not affect the duration or pattern of EEG seizure activity.[317]

Anticonvulsive Actions

Although the CNS effects of local anesthetic agents are usually considered to be undesirable, the depressant action on the CNS has proven to be of therapeutic value in certain clinical conditions.[341] Studies in animals have demonstrated that procaine, lidocaine, and prilocaine are capable of preventing various forms of experimentally induced convulsions. Infiltration of exposed scalp wound margins with 30 mg of lidocaine or 60 mg of procaine significantly increased the threshold for electrically induced cortical after-discharges in cats.[342,343] Lidocaine also exhibited anticonvulsant activity in cats with penicillin-induced epileptogenic foci[344] and in mice with audiogenic seizures and electrically induced convulsions,[345,346] while procaine was shown to protect mice against electroshock-induced convulsions.[347] Most of the clinically useful local anesthetic agents demonstrate anticonvulsant activity, and a correlation has been observed between the anticonvulsive and intrinsic anesthetic potency of the various compounds (Fig. 6-3).[341]

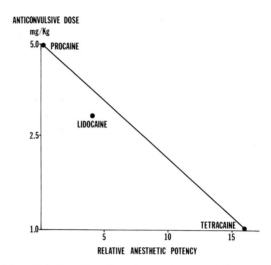

Fig. 6-3. Relationship of anticonvulsant activity of various local anesthetic agents to their relative anesthetic potency.

        In general, the anticonvulsant activity of local anesthetic agents occurs at doses and blood levels considerably lower than the dose and blood level associated with seizure activity. Julien has correlated the arterial blood levels of lidocaine with the antiepileptic and seizure-inducing properties of this agent in cats in whom epileptiform activity was produced by intracortical injections of penicillin. A marked anti-epileptic effect was observed at lidocaine blood levels of 0.5–4.0 μg/ml. When the blood level of lidocaine reached 4.5–7.0 μg/ml, signs of increased cortical irritability again were observed. At blood levels in excess of 7.5 μg/ml, seizure activity reoccurred.

        Clinically, procaine and lidocaine have been employed to prevent and/or reduce the duration of electrically induced seizures in patients.[348,355] The anticonvulsant dose of both agents was found to be lower than the dose which caused seizure activity, e.g., 5–11 mg/kg was the anticonvulsant dose of lidocaine, whereas 16 mg/kg produced a seizure state.[348] Procaine and, particularly, lidocaine also have been utilized to terminate or decrease the duration of grand mal or petit mal seizures.[341] Presumably, the mechanism of the anticonvulsant action of local anesthetic agents in epileptic patients involves a depression of hyperexcitable cortical neurons.

CARDIOVASCULAR EFFECTS

Regional anesthesia can produce profound changes in the cardiovascular system due to the direct effect of local anesthetic agents on cardiac tissue and peripheral vasculature and also indirectly by conduction blockade of autonomic nerve fibers that regulate cardiac and peripheral vascular functions.

Direct Action of Local Anesthetic Agents

CARDIAC EFFECTS

Much information has been obtained concerning the cardiac effects of local anesthetic agents, particularly, lidocaine, because of the clinical use of this drug for the treatment of ventricular arrhythmias. Detailed studies concerning the effect of lidocaine on the electrophysiological properties of isolated cardiac tissue have revealed a consistent sequence of events as the dose and subsequent blood level of local anesthetic agent are increased[349-351] (Table 39). At doses and blood levels of lidocaine that are nontoxic, but sufficient for antiarrhythmic activity, the only discernable electrophysiological effects observed were a prolongation or abolition of the phase of slow depolarization during diastole (phase 4 depolarization) in Purkinje fibers and a shortening of the action potential duration (APD) and of the effective refractory period (ERP). However, the ratio of effective refractory period to action potential duration (ERP/APD) increased both in Purkinje fibers and in ventricu-

Table 39

CARDIOVASCULAR ALTERATIONS WITH PROGRESSIVE INCREASES IN LOCAL ANESTHETIC DOSE (LIDOCAINE)

Dose µg/kg/min	Blood levels µg/ml	Electrophysiological effects		Hemodynamic effects	
		Cellular change	Surface changes	Cardiac	Peripheral Vascular
20-50	2-5	↑ Phase IV Depolarization ↓ APD ↓ ERP ↑ ERP/APD ↑ Conduction velocity PF-VM	—	—	—
50-75	5-10	↓ Phase 0 Depolarization ↓ AP amplitude ↓ Conduction velocity	↑ PR interval ↑ QRS duration Sinus bradycardia	↑ End-diastolic volume ↑ Intraventricular pressure ↓ Myocardial contraction ↓ Cardiac output	Vasodilation ↓ Blood pressure
>75	>10	↓↓ Phase 0 Depolarization ↓↓ AP amplitude ↓↓ Conduction velocity	↓↓ PR interval ↓↓ QRS duration Sinus bradycardia AV block Aystole	↓↓ End-diastolic volume ↓↓ Intraventricular pressure ↓↓ Myocardial contraction ↓↓ Cardiac output	↓↓ Blood pressure Circulatory collapse

lar muscle. No change was evident in resting potential, rate of rise of the action potential, or action potential amplitude. The conduction velocity in Purkinje fibers was minimally altered, whereas conduction at the junction between Purkinje fibers and ventricular muscle was enhanced. Toxic concentrations of lidocaine resulted in a decrease in maximum rate of depolarization of Purkinje fibers and ventricular muscle, a decrease in amplitude of the action potential, and a marked reduction in conduction velocity. However, even at a lidocaine concentration of 50 μg/ml, the resting potential remained unchanged. In general, local anesthetic agents appear to modify in a similar fashion the electrophysiological events in cardiac tissue and in peripheral nerve, i.e., the rate of rise of the various phases of depolarization is reduced as the concentration of local anesthetic agents is increased with no appreciable alteration in resting membrane potential and no marked prolongation of the repolarization phase. Electrophysiological studies of the heart in intact dogs and man essentially reflect the findings observed in isolated cardiac tissue.[352-355] Doses of lidocaine that are considered nontoxic produce minimal changes in intraatrial, intraventricular, and atrioventricular conduction, absolute refractory period, and diastolic threshold. As the dose of lidocaine is increased, a prolongation of conduction time through various portions of the heart as well as an increase in diastolic threshold occurs. These changes are reflected in the electrocardiogram as an increased PR interval and QRS duration and decreased automaticity, as shown by sinus bradycardia and, finally, cardiac arrest, i.e., asystole, when extremely high local anesthetic blood levels are obtained.

The electrophysiological changes produced by lidocaine are related to effects on ion flux across the membrane of the cardiac cell. Slow depolarization during diastole, i.e., phase 4 depolarization, is a function of the gradual decrease in potassium permeability across the cardiac cell membrane. Studies on isolated cardiac tissue in which ion flux measurements have been made prior to and during treatment with lidocaine have revealed an increase in potassium efflux.[356] This efflux of potassium ions may be responsible for the prolongation or abolition of the slow phase of depolarization. The increase in potassium efflux occurred in ventricular muscle, but not in atrial muscle treated with lidocaine. This observation correlates well with the antiarrhythmic efficacy of lidocaine in clinical practice, i.e., lidocaine is effective in the treatment of cardiac arrhythmias of ventricular origin, but is considerably less efficacious in controlling atrial arrhythmias. Higher doses of lidocaine were associated with a decrease in the rate of phase 0 depolarization, which presumably reflects an inhibition of sodium conductance similar to the situation in peripheral nerve leading to conduction blockade. Detailed cardiac electrophysiological studies have not been conducted with other local anesthetic agents. However, mepivacaine, prilocaine, and bupivacaine also demonstrate antiarrhythmic activity in various animal models.[357,358]

The effect of local anesthetic agents on the mechanical activity of cardiac muscle has also been extensively studied. The results in animals are somewhat contradictory, since at relatively low doses a decrease, an increase, and no change in myocardial contractility or cardiac output have been reported.[359,360] As the dosage of local anesthetic agent is increased to toxic levels, these drugs do exert a direct negative inotropic action on cardiac muscle.[361,362] The relative myocardial depressant action of various local anesthetic agents is correlated with their intrinsic anesthetic potency.[361] For example, the anesthetic potency and myocardial toxicity of lidocaine in relation to procaine have both been reported to be approximately four to one (Fig. 6-4). In general, the hemodynamic effects of local anesthetic agents in man correlate quite well with the results obtained from animal studies.[352,363-368] At lidocaine doses and blood levels considered nontoxic, but still sufficient for antiarrhythmic activity, no alterations in myocardial contractility, diastolic volume, intraventricular pressure, and cardiac output are usually observed. A progressive increase in dose and blood levels results in decreased myocardial contractility, increased diastolic volume, decreased intraventricular

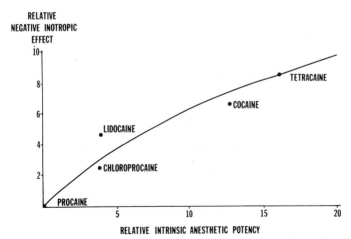

Fig. 6-4. Relative negative inotropic effect and intrinsic anesthetic potency of various local anesthetic agents.

pressure, and decreased cardiac output (Table 39). The usual doses of the various local anesthetic agents employed for regional anesthesia result in peak blood levels which generally are not associated with a cardiodepressant effect. However, the inadvertent rapid intravenous administration of a local anesthetic agent or the administration of excessive doses may cause a significant decrease in myocardial contractility and cardiac output, contributing to circulatory collapse.

PERIPHERAL VASCULAR EFFECTS

Local anesthetic agents tend to produce a biphasic effect on vascular smooth muscle (Table 40). In vitro studies have demonstrated that, at low concentration, all agents studied stimulated spontaneous myogenic contractions in preparations such as the isolated rat portal vein and, in some cases, augmented the basal tone of the vascular smooth muscle preparation.[263,369-371] The increase in the height of spontaneous smooth muscle contractility did not appear to be correlated with the anesthetic potency of the various compounds. For example, prilocaine produced the greatest enhancement of myogenic activity while etidocaine was least effective. Prilocaine, mepivacaine, and procaine also produced the greatest increase in basal tone, whereas minimal changes were seen with lidocaine, tetracaine, bupivacaine, and etidocaine[263] (Table 40).

In vivo studies have confirmed this initial stimulatory effect of local anesthetic agents on vascular smooth muscle. Intra-arterial administration of mepivacaine in human volunteers produced a decrease in forearm blood flow without altering arterial pressure, which is indicative of an increase in peripheral vascular resistance. Similar studies with lidocaine also showed an increased tone of capacitance vessels with less consistent effects on resistance vessels.[372] Moreover, in animal preparations in which vascular tone had been

Table 40

BIPHASIC PERIPHERAL VASCULAR EFFECT OF VARIOUS LOCAL ANESTHETIC AGENTS

AGENT	ISOLATED RAT PORTAL VEIN % Increase (constriction)		CANINE FEMORAL BLOOD FLOW % Increase (dilation)
	Spontaneous contractions	Basal tone	
LIDOCAINE	173	68	25
MEPIVACAINE	228	162	36
PRILOCAINE	293	163	42
TETRACAINE	237	82	38
BUPIVACAINE	184	37	45
ETIDOCAINE	147	—	44

reduced by alpha-adrenergic blockade or spinal section, mepivacaine and procaine were found to produce an increase in hind-limb vascular resistance.[373,374]

An increase in the dose of local anesthetic agent administered was associated with an inhibition of myogenic activity in vitro and vasodilation in vivo.[263,266] Lidocaine, mepivacaine, prilocaine, and tetracaine were all found to produce an increased blood flow in the hind limb of dogs and cats following intraarterial administration.[110,266] Similar studies in man have also shown that lidocaine, mepivacaine, and bupivacaine caused vasodilation and an increase in forearm blood flow.[264] A comparison of the peripheral vascular effects of various local anesthetic agents revealed a 25% to 45% increase in canine femoral blood flow following the intraarterial administration of 1 ml of 1% lidocaine, mepivacaine, tetracaine, prilocaine, etidocaine, and bupivacaine (Table 40).[263] Although no correlation was observed between peripheral vascular effects and anesthetic potency, a relationship existed between duration of anesthesia and vasodilation produced by these various agents. At 5 minutes following the intraarterial administration of lidocaine, mepivacaine, and prilocaine, femoral blood flow had returned to normal, whereas those agents that possess a longer duration of local anesthetic activity, i.e., bupivacaine, etidocaine, and tetracaine continued to show a 14% to 30% increase in femoral arterial flow.[263]

Cocaine is the only local anesthetic agent that produces systemic vasoconstriction at doses commonly employed for regional anesthetic procedures.[266] Direct blood flow studies in dogs have revealed that the initial effect of cocaine is one of vasodilation, followed by a prolonged period of vasoconstriction. As indicated previously, this vasoconstrictor action appeared related to an inhibition of the uptake of norepinephrine into tissue-binding sites.[267] This property has not been demonstrated with other drugs, such as lidocaine and mepivacaine.[375]

The biphasic peripheral vascular effect of local anesthetic agents may be related to changes in smooth muscle concentrations of calcium. A competitive antagonism exists between local anesthetic drugs and calcium ions in smooth muscle.[376,377] Local anesthetic compounds may displace Ca^{++} from membrane-binding sites, which results in diffusion of this ion into the smooth muscle cytoplasm. Such an increase in cytoplasmic calcium concentration will stimulate the interaction between contractile proteins leading to an increase in myogenic contractility, i.e., vasoconstriction. Ultimately, the displacement of calcium by increasing doses of local anesthetic agents will decrease both the cytoplasmic Ca^{++} concentration and the interaction between the contractile protein elements of smooth muscle, which results in a state of muscle relaxation, i.e., vasodilation.

In general, the sequence of cardiovascular events observed following a progressive increase in local anesthetic dosage can be summarized as follows: at doses of local anesthetic agents that produce nontoxic blood levels, either a slight increase or no change in blood pressure occurs. The slight increase in blood pressure is probably related to (a) an increase in cardiac output and heart rate which is believed due to an enhancement of sympathetic activity and (b) a direct vasoconstriction of certain peripheral vascular beds. Blood levels of local anesthetic agents approaching toxic concentrations cause hypotension as a result of peripheral vasodilation resulting from a direct relaxant effect on peripheral vascular smooth muscle. A further elevation of local anesthetic blood levels produces a decreased myocardial contractility, which results in a fall in cardiac output. This combination of reduced peripheral vascular resistance and cardiac output leads to profound hypotension. Finally, at lethal blood levels of local anesthetic agents, cardiovascular collapse ensues due to massive peripheral vasodilation, marked reduction in myocardial contractility, and slowed heart rate, which ultimately results in cardiac arrest.

The direct circulatory actions of local anesthetic agents may be altered by the concomitant administration of other drugs. As indicated previously, nontoxic doses of local anesthetic agents may produce either minimal changes in blood pressure or may have a stimulatory effect on the myocardium and peripheral vasculature. The use of CNS depressant drugs such as general anesthetic agents and ganglionic blocking agents will block the positive inotropic action of lidocaine that is mediated via the sympathetic nervous system.[378, 379] Therefore, nondepressant doses of a local anesthetic agent may result in cardiovascular depression when administered in the presence of barbiturates or other drugs that inhibit CNS activity. Diazepam, which can effectively prevent the CNS toxicity of local anesthetic agents, does not modify the circulatory depression of these drugs.[380]

Indirect Effect of Local Anesthetic Agents

The cardiovascular changes due to the direct effect of the local anesthetic agent itself should be distinguished from alterations secondary to the regional anesthetic procedure performed. Central neural blocks of the lumbar epidural or subarachnoid type are frequently associated with a fall in systemic blood pressure.[222, 381-383] For example,

Moore and his co-workers reported hypotension in 38% to 45% of patients following spinal or epidural anesthesia.[222] Subarachnoid anesthesia to the T_5 level caused a decrease in stroke volume, cardiac output, and peripheral vascular resistance, which undoubtedly accounts for the rather high rate of hypotension.[384] Since the doses used for spinal anesthesia are quite small, such cardiovascular changes during subarachnoid anesthesia appear related solely to the sympathetic blockade produced by this procedure, rather than a direct effect of the local anesthetic agent. Hypotension may also occur following epidural anesthesia, but the mechanism appears to be more complex. The degree of hypotension following peridural blockade is related, in part, to the level of anesthesia, the local anesthetic agent, the concomitant use of vasoconstrictor drugs, and the status of the patient[385] (Fig. 6-5). For example, Bonica and associates reported that epidural anesthesia extending to the first thoracic segment or higher was associated with a fall in mean arterial blood pressure of 16%, a decrease in total peripheral

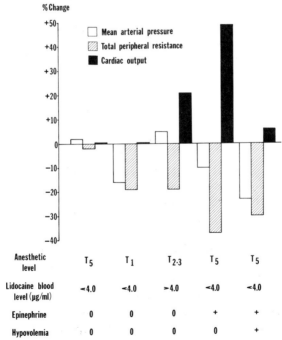

Fig. 6-5. Cardiovascular effects of epidural anesthesia as influenced by analgesic dermatomal level, anesthetic blood level, epinephrine, and presence of hyporvolemia.

resistance (TPR) of 18%, and little change in cardiac output.[386] However, analgesia to T_4 or below failed to produce a significant change in blood pressure, peripheral resistance, or cardiac output.[386] These differences were related to the extent of the sympathetic blockade. T_1 blocks resulted in a significant increase in both upper- and lower-limb blood flow and a fall in TPR, which indicates widespread sympathetic blockade and peripheral vasodilation. T_4 blockade produced an increase in lower-limb blood flow, but a fall in upper-limb flow and little change in TPR, which suggests a compensatory vasoconstriction in the upper half of the body.

Relatively large doses of local anesthetic agents are employed for epidural anesthesia. As indicated in Chapter 5, local analgesic drugs are well absorbed from the epidural space. For example, lidocaine blood levels of 4–7 μg/ml occurred in some of the subjects involved in the epidural study conducted by Bonica, Berges, and Morikawa.[386] In these subjects, a fall in TPR was offset by an increase in cardiac output such that little change in mean arterial blood pressure occurred. The increased cardiac output was believed due to a direct effect of lidocaine on the vasomotor center in the CNS. The use of excessive amounts of local anesthetic drug for regional anesthesia will result in blood levels that may produce direct cardiac and peripheral vascular depression, exaggerating the hypotensive state caused by sympathetic blockade.

Central neural blockade may also cause a decrease in renal plasma flow and hepatic blood flow.[387,388] Since amide-type local anesthetic drugs are metabolized in the liver and excreted via the kidney, decreases in renal and hepatic blood flow will retard the clearance of these agents and possibly augment their direct cardiovascular effects.

The specific local anesthetic agent employed can influence the changes in cardiovascular function produced by the regional anesthetic procedure. A comparison of drugs of different inherent anesthetic duration, i.e., lidocaine and etidocaine, in epidural analgesia revealed that the magnitude of cardiovascular changes was similar for the two agents, but the duration of hypotension following etidocaine blockade was significantly prolonged.[211] This prolonged hypotensive action was directly related to the longer duration of epidural anesthesia and sympathetic blockade produced by etidocaine.

Anesthetic solutions employed for epidural analgesia frequently contain a vasoconstrictor drug, usually epinephrine, which influences the circulatory changes associated with the anesthetic procedure. Epidural blockade to the T_5 level with plain lidocaine produced a 5% to 10% change in cardiac output, peripheral resistance, and arterial pressure. In contrast, lidocaine with epinephrine resulted in a 49% increase in cardiac output, 37% decrease in total peripheral resistance, and a 10% decrease in mean arterial pressure. The marked increase in cardiac output and decrease in TPR were ascribed to the beta-adrenergic receptor-stimulating effect of absorbed epinephrine.[389]

The physiological status of the patient also influences the circulatory changes following regional anesthesia. The use of lidocaine-epinephrine solutions to induce epidural analgesia in hypovolemic subjects caused a 23% decrease in arterial pressure compared to a 10% fall in normovolemic volunteers. This difference was due to the absence of a compensatory increase in cardiac output in the hypovolemic subjects. Epidural administration of plain lidocaine in the presence of hypovolemia produced signs of severe cardiovascular depression which were believed related to a greater myocardial uptake of lidocaine, leading to a significant decrease in cardiac contractility.[390]

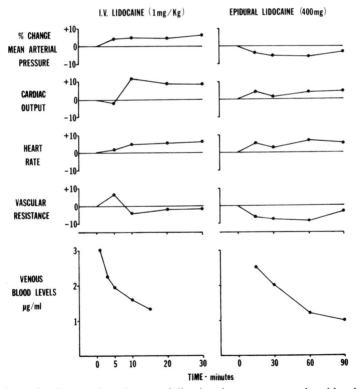

Fig. 6-6. Cardiovascular changes following intravenous and epidural administration of lidocaine.

The circulatory effect of other forms of regional anesthesia has also been studied.[391] Sciatic-femoral blocks utilizing either 125 mg of bupivacaine or 500 mg of lidocaine with epinephrine 1: 200,000 caused a decrease in peripheral resistance, an increase in cardiac output and heart rate, and no change in blood pressure. The increase in cardiac output may be reflex in origin or may be related to absorbed epinephrine and the CNS-stimulating effect of the local anesthetic agent, since lidocaine exerted a significantly greater positive inotropic action than bupivacaine.

The direct cardiovascular effect of local anesthetic agents and the circulatory alterations due to the regional anesthetic procedure can be compared in the following manner (Fig. 6-6): the blood level of lidocaine following the administration of 400 mg of this agent into the lumbar epidural space is similar to that produced by the IV injection of 1 mg/kg of lidocaine. However, the cardiovascular effects are quite different. Little or no change in blood pressure, peripheral vascular resistance, cardiac output, and heart rate occurs following the IV administration of 1 mg/kg lidocaine. On the other hand, epidural anesthesia results in a significant fall in arterial blood pressure, due primarily to a decrease in peripheral vascular resistance, with little or no change in cardiac output, and a slight rise in heart rate. These cardiovascular effects are obviously due to sympathetic blockade and a subsequent reduction in peripheral vascular tone rather than a direct vasodilator effect of the local anesthetic agent.

RESPIRATORY EFFECTS

Local anesthetic agents exert a biphasic effect on respiration. At subtoxic doses, a direct relaxant effect on bronchial smooth muscle may offset any depressant action on CNS respiratory centers.[392] Intravenously administered mepivacaine and bupivacaine in man did not produce a significant alteration on pCO_2, pO_2, pH, or oxygen saturation.[393] Excessive amounts of local anesthetic agents can cause respiratory arrest due to their generalized CNS depressant action.

Certain regional anesthetic procedures may be associated with alterations in pulmonary function. Thoracic epidural anesthesia extending from T_2-T_{12} produced a significant decrease in various pulmonary function tests such as FVC and $FEV_{1.0}$, whereas minimal changes occurred following thoracolumbar epidural anesthesia from T_4-L_4.[394,395] Subarachnoid or epidural blockade to the T_5 level did not result in any deleterious change in blood gas tensions.[384]

Postoperative respiratory function is frequently abnormal in patients undergoing upper-abdominal procedures. Comparisons of the pulmonary status of patients treated with either parenteral opiates or epidural analgesia for postoperative pain relief have demonstrated that epidural nerve blocks may be superior to narcotic analgesia in reducing the degree of postoperative pulmonary dysfunction which can lead to hypoxemia.[396,397]

Numerous studies have been conducted to evaluate fetal acid-base status following epidural or paracervical blocks for obstetrical anesthesia. Minimal alterations in the acid-base status of the fetus have been associated with the use of a variety of local anesthetic drugs for obstetrical analgesic procedures.[281,284,286,398] However, other factors, such as maternal hypotension associated with the anesthetic technique or addition of epinephrine 1:200,000 to the local anesthetic solution, may cause changes in the acid-base status of the fetus.[284,399]

MISCELLANEOUS EFFECTS

Other pharmacological actions ascribed to local anesthetic drugs include ganglionic blockade,[400] neuromuscular blockade,[401] anticholinergic,[402] antihistaminic,[403] and antibacterial activity.[404]

The effect of local anesthetic agents on neuromuscular transmission has been studied extensively. Procaine, lidocaine, mepivacaine, prilocaine, and bupivacaine have been demonstrated to inhibit in vitro myoneural junction preparations and to block neuromuscular transmission in man.[401,405-408] Although localized neuromuscular paralysis occurs following the intra-arterial injection of local anesthetic drugs in man, minimal alterations in neuromuscular activity have been observed when these agents were administered intravenously.[401,408]

Local anesthetic neuromuscular blockade may involve either pre- or postjunctional structures. Galindo ascribed the depressant action of procaine at the myoneural junction to an inhibition of the prejunctional motor-nerve terminal.[407] Other investigators have reported that local anesthetic agents either decrease the sensitivity of the postjunctional motor end plate to acetylcholine or block the depolarizing action of acetylcholine on the motor end plate.[401,405,406] Measurements of ionic conductances across the end-plate membrane have demonstrated that procaine exerts a profound inhibitory effect on sodium flux, which suggests that the basic action of local anesthetic agents is similar for all excitable membranes, i.e., a block of sodium channels in the cell membrane.[409]

Drug Interaction

The miscellaneous actions of local anesthetic drugs do not appear to be clinically relevant when the agents are employed alone. However, the interaction of local anesthetic agents with other types of drugs may be clinically significant. This is a particular problem in anesthesiology, since patients frequently receive multiple medications.[410] For example, the neuromuscular blocking action of local anesthetic agents alone is clinically irrelevant, but such agents can significantly enhance the action of both depolarizing and nondepolarizing myoneural blockers.[401,408] It has been demonstrated in dogs and man that the duration of apnea produced by succinylcholine or curare can be considerably prolonged by lidocaine.[411,412] As shown previously, premedication with CNS depressant drugs such as barbiturates can decrease the CNS toxicity, but may potentiate the cardiodepressant effect of local anesthetic agents. Other agents such as iproniazid, isoniazid, chloramphenicol, promethazine, and meperidine have been reported to enhance or prolong the convulsive action of local anesthetic drugs in animals.[413,414]

The concomitant use of local anesthetic agents and other drugs that share common metabolic pathways may cause adverse effects in patients. Prolonged apnea may occur if succinylcholine and the procaine-like ester drugs are employed together, since plasma pseudocholinesterase is required for the hydrolysis of both types of drugs.[292] Inducers of hepatic microsomal enzyme systems may alter the rate of metabolism of the lidocaine-like amide agents,[415] as indicated by an increase in the rate at which metabolites of lidocaine are formed in phenobarbital-treated dogs.[416]

TOXICOLOGICAL EFFECTS

Allergy

Most investigators believe that true allergic reactions to local anesthetic agents are extremely rare.[182,417,418] However, reports of suspected allergic, hypersensitivity, or anaphylactic responses to local anesthetic compounds appear periodically in the literature.[419-421] Usually, the diagnosis of such reactions is made when no obvious explanation is available for an adverse effect in a patient exposed to a local anesthetic drug. The ester derivatives of para-aminobenzoic acid, such as procaine, were responsible for most of the dermal allergic phenomena which were usually experienced by members of the dental profession. Such reports have been infrequent with the amide-type local analgesic compounds. True allergy requires the formation of an antibody to an antigenic substance. To date, no evidence is available that antibodies are formed in response to a challenge by an amide-type local anesthetic drug. Aldrete and Johnson used the technique of intracutaneous testing to study patients with and without a presumptive history of local anesthetic allergy.[422] Positive skin reactions were observed in 25 of 60 patients in the nonallergic group. In all cases, the cutaneous reaction followed injection of an ester-type local anesthetic agent such as procaine, tetracaine, and chloroprocaine. No reactions were observed after treatment with the amide-type agents, lidocaine, mepivacaine, or prilocaine. Eleven patients had a history of alleged local anesthetic allergy. In eight of these cases, a positive skin reaction to procaine, tetracaine, or chloroprocaine was produced, but no positive skin response was seen with lidocaine, mepivacaine, or prilocaine. In none of these subjects were signs of systemic anaphylaxis observed. Solutions of the amide-type local anesthetic agents may contain as a preservative, methylparaben, whose structure is similar to para-aminobenzoic acid. Some patients presumed to be allergic to lidocaine have shown a positive skin response to methylparaben, but not to lidocaine itself.[423]

It is obviously difficult to study in a controlled fashion anaphylactic-type reactions. The low rate of adverse events reported in epidemiological studies involving local or regional anesthesia suggests that systemic anaphylaxis to local anesthetic agents must be quite rare.[424] Undoubtedly, anaphylactic-type reactions may occur with any drug. However, any unusual adverse response should be thoroughly investigated before a presumptive diagnosis of anaphylaxis is made. This may be particularly difficult with local anesthetic agents, since the circulatory crisis of true systemic anaphylaxis may be indistinguishable from the state of cardiovascular collapse that can follow an excessive dose, rapid absorption from a highly vascular site, or an inadvertent IV injection of a local anesthetic agent. Moreover, the addition of vasoconstrictor agents, particularly epinephrine, to local anesthetic solutions makes it difficult to differentiate the pharmacological effects of an excess level of catecholamines from the symptoms of anaphylaxis. Finally, the potential interaction of concomitant medications in anesthesia can obscure the differential diagnosis of adverse systemic reactions.

Local Tissue Toxicity

The effect of local anesthetic agents on various tissue cells has been investigated to determine their potential local irritation. Local anesthetic agents cause hemolysis of red blood cells in direct relationship to the intrinsic anesthetic potency of the specific compound.[425] However, the concentrations of local anesthetic agents that produce red-blood-cell hemolysis in vitro are considerably higher than in vivo concentrations achieved clinically. The inhibition of leukocytic aggregation and the adherence of leukocytes to the intima of blood vessels at anesthetic blood concentrations which are achieved during regional anesthesia has been reported.[426] The clinical significance of these findings are, as yet, unclear.

The use of local anesthetic agents in the concentrations that are clinically available has not been shown to produce localized nerve damage.[427, 428] Studies on the isolated frog sciatic nerve have revealed that concentrations of procaine, cocaine, tetracaine, and dibucaine required to produce irreversible conduction blockade are far in excess of those used clinically.[425] A comparison of lidocaine, tetracaine, or etidocaine administered subdurally in rabbits revealed histopathological spinal cord changes following the use of 4% tetracaine, which is considerably greater than the concentrations (0.25–1%) employed for spinal anesthesia in man.[429] Fink and co-workers have described an inhibitory effect of local anesthetic agents on rapid axonal transport in the rat vagus nerve.[430] This change in rapid axonal transport is not associated with changes in the ultrastructure of peripheral nerve, and the clinical significance of these findings is not apparent at present.

It has also been suggested that preservatives in local anesthetic solutions may cause neurotoxicity. MacDonald and Watkins reported that the concentration of chemical preservatives in spinal anesthetic solutions was insufficient to cause paralysis.[431] Studies have been conducted to evaluate the neurotoxic effects of methylparaben, a common antibacterial preservative in multiple-dose local anesthetic containers. Methylparaben with and without lidocaine was administered into the subarachnoid space of rabbits and failed to produce any histopathological evidence of neurotoxicity.[432]

Several studies have been performed which indicate that local anesthetic agents can cause histological changes in skeletal muscle.[427, 428, 433] Skeletal muscle changes have been observed with most of the clinically used local anesthetic compounds such as lidocaine, mepivacaine, prilocaine, bupivacaine, and etidocaine. In general, the more potent, longer-acting compounds appear to cause a greater degree of localized skeletal muscle damage than the less potent, shorter-acting agents. This effect on skeletal muscle is reversible and muscle regeneration occurs rapidly and is complete within 2 weeks following the injection of local anesthetic agents.[427, 428] These changes in skeletal muscle have not been correlated with any overt clinical signs of local irritation.

However, an increase in blood levels of creatine phosphokinase (CPK) have been reported following the intramuscular administration of lidocaine, which is indicative of skeletal muscle damage.[434]

Systemic Toxicity

As described previously, local anesthetic toxicity involves essentially the central nervous system and the cardiovascular system. Adverse reactions are usually due to a rapid inadvertent intravenous injection, administration into a highly vascular anatomical site, or administration of an excessive amount of local anesthetic drug. In each instance, a high blood level of local anesthetic agent is achieved. Adverse reactions to a local anesthetic agent usually proceed in the following manner: (a) premonitory CNS symptoms such as dizziness, ringing in the ears, vague sensation of light headedness, nystagmus, fine skeletal muscle twitching of face and digits; (b) overt convulsions of a clonic and tonic nature; (c) CNS depression in which seizure activity terminates and respiratory efforts become shallow and, ultimately, cease; (d) fall in systemic blood pressure; and (e) a progressive bradycardia leading ultimately to cardiac arrest. Rapid achievement of an extremely high anesthetic blood level may produce respiratory depression and cardiovascular collapse without the usual signs and symptoms of CNS excitation.

Treatment of systemic local anesthetic reactions requires a recognition of the warning symptoms described above and knowledge of the organ systems affected by overdosage of local anesthetic agents. Initial treatment should be directed toward ensuring the presence of a patent airway and providing a source of oxygen. Maintenance of an adequate respiratory exchange will often suffice in the treatment of the early stages of acute systemic reactions. The occurrence of convulsive activity requires the use of CNS depressant agents to control the generalized seizures. Intravenous diazepam and short-acting barbiturates have been shown to be effective in aborting local anesthetic-induced seizures. Short-acting neuromuscular blocking agents, such as succinylcholine, have also been utilized to inhibit overt convulsions and to permit a more adequate control of respiration. However, neuromuscular blocking agents do not affect the increased electrical activity of the brain, so that CNS depressant drugs are still required to control the state of CNS excitation, and ventilation should be assisted until such time as the patient is capable of spontaneous respiration. Respiratory depression is usually indicative of an extremely high anesthetic blood level. As the anesthetic blood level declines, the patient may reenter a phase of CNS excitation and convulsive activity may reoccur.

Signs and symptoms of cardiovascular collapse require treatment with vasopressor or positive inotropic agents in order to support the circulation. Since vasodilation is usually responsible for the initial fall in blood pressure, vasopressor agents such as phenylephrine and methoxamine, which act predominantly on the peripheral vasculature may be preferable. Later stages of circulatory collapse involve a decrease in myocardial contractility and cardiac output, and the use of vasopressor agents such as ephedrine or norepinephrine, which possess a positive inotropic action, may be desirable to constrict the peripheral vasculature and to increase cardiac contractility.

Knowledge of therapeutic methods to control the systemic toxicity of local anesthetic agents is essential. However, most adverse reactions can be avoided by observing certain precautions that involve a knowledge of the local anesthetic agent employed, the regional anesthetic procedure to be performed, and the clinical status of the patient. The selection of a proper anesthetic dose requires an awareness of the inherent anesthetic potency of a specific agent and the selective rate of systemic absorption from the injection site in order to avert the accidental administration of an overdose. Care and skill in performance of the anesthetic procedure are necessary to prevent an inadvertent intravascular injection. The clinical status of the patient will dictate the choice and dose of local anesthetic agent. For example, the clearance of local anesthetic agents is decreased in patients with cardiac failure and poor hepatic perfusion, which necessitates the use of lower dosages. Patients with advanced hepatic or renal disease are more vulnerable to the toxic effects of amide-type agents, whereas the presence of atypical pseudocholinesterase may enhance the potential for systemic reactions to ester-type drugs.

In general, local anesthetic agents possess a lower therapeutic ratio than normally would be considered clinically desirable. However, these agents are usually administered into a circumscribed area of the body by trained clinicians, so that the frequency of adverse reactions associated with local anesthetic drugs is remarkably low. Retrospective and prospective studies of epidural and spinal anesthesia involving more than 10,000 patients per study with a variety of anesthetic agents demonstrated a 0.3% to 1.5% frequency of complications associated with the anesthetic procedure.[218,435] A review of the world literature on epidural anesthesia by Dawkins in 1969 revealed a 0.2% frequency of toxic reactions in more than 60,000 cases.[424] Since some of the adverse events reported in these surveys are attributable to the anesthetic technique itself or factors unrelated to the anesthetic agent, the incidence of true local anesthetic-induced reactions must be extremely low. Therefore, local anesthesia provides a safe and efficacious method of preventing or alleviating pain in circumscribed anatomical areas. However, the judicious use of regional anesthesia requires knowledge of the pharmacological properties of the specific agents employed, technical skill in the performance of the various nerve-blocking procedures, and a thorough evaluation of the patient's clinical status.

SUMMARY

1. Local anesthetic agents may exert pharmacological actions other than peripheral nerve blockade. The central nervous system and cardiovascular system are particularly susceptible to the effect of local anesthetic drugs.
2. As the dosage and blood level of local anesthetic agents are progressively increased, an initial excitatory CNS effect occurs followed by a state of generalized CNS depression. The convulsive action of local anesthetic agents is related to an inhibition of inhibitory cortical neurons such that facilitory pathways act in an unopposed fashion leading to seizure activity. At higher anesthetic dose levels an inhibition of both inhibitory and facilitory neurons causes generalized CNS depression.
3. Local anesthetic-induced changes in the cardiovascular system are characterized initially by an increase in peripheral vascular resistance due to a direct effect on peripheral vascular smooth muscle and an increase in cardiac output due indirectly to an action on the CNS. The predominant cardiovascular effects of high doses of local anesthetic agents include systemic hypotension due to a generalized vasodilation and a decrease in myocardial contractility, leading to a fall in cardiac output. Sinus bradycardia and, ultimately, cardiac arrest can occur due to the use of lethal doses of local anesthetic agents.
4. Respiration is unaffected by local anesthetic agents until doses causing overt CNS toxicity are achieved. The miscellaneous actions of local anesthetic drugs are usually not clinically relevant unless they are employed in combination with other agents such as neuromuscular blockers.
5. True allergic reactions to local anesthetic agents are extremely rare and are mainly referable to the use of the procaine-like ester compounds. Certain preservatives in local anesthetic solutions such as methylparaben may also cause allergic reactions.

6. The local tissue toxicity of regional anesthetic agents is limited primarily to skeletal muscle and is spontaneously reversible. No cytotoxic effects have been observed in nerves exposed to the normal concentrations of clinically available agents.

7. Systemic toxicity is usually due to an inadvertent intravascular injection, administration into highly vascular sites, or use of an excessive dose. Treatment consists of maintenance of a patent airway, adequate ventilation, use of anticonvulsant agents, such as diazepam or barbiturates, to control seizures, and vasopressor drugs to support circulation if hypotension should occur.

References

1. de Jong RH: Physiology and Pharmacology of Local Anesthesia. Springfield, Illinois, Charles C Thomas, 1970, p 5
2. Moréno y Maiz T: Recherches Chimiques et Physiologiques sur l'Erythroxylum Coca du Pérou et la Cocaine. Paris, Leclerc, 1868, pp 77 and 79
3. Koller C: Lancet 2:990, 1884
4. Ritsert E: Pharm Ztg 37:427, 1892
5. Braun H: Dent Med Wochschr 31:1667, 1905
6. Einhorn A, Uhlfelder E: Ann Chem 371:131, 1909
7. Fussganger R, Schaumann O: Arch Exp Pathol Pharmackol 160:53, 1931
8. Foldes FF, McNall PG: Anesthesiology 13:287, 1952
9. Löfgren N: Studies on Local Anesthetics. Xylocaine: a New Synthetic Drug. Stockholm, Hoeggstroms, 1948
10. Takman BH, Boyes RN, Vassallo HG: Local Anesthetics Medicinal Chemistry, ed 4. New York, John Wiley & Sons, Inc, 1974
11. Löfgren N, Tegnér C: Acta Chem Scand 14:486, 1960
12. Adams HJ, Kronberg GH, Takman BH: J Pharmacol Sci 61:1829, 1972
13. Ekenstam B, Egner B, Pettersson G: Acta Chem Scand 11:1183, 1957
14. Ulfendahl HR: Acta Anaesthesiol Scand 1:81, 1957
15. Henn F, Brattsand R: Acta Anaesthesiol Scand, (Suppl) 21, p 9, 1966
16. Goto T, Kishi Y, Takahashi S, Hirata Y: Tetrahedron 21:2059, 1965
17. Schantz EJ, Ghazarossian VE, Schnoes HK, Strong FM, Springer JP, Pezzanite JO, Clardy J: J Am Chem Soc 97:1238, 1975
18. Kao CY: Pharmacol Rev 18:997, 1966
19. Schantz EJ: Ann NY Acad Sci 90:843, 1960
20. Truant AP, Takman B: Anesth Analg 38:478, 1959
21. Tucker GT, Boyes RN, Bridenbaugh PO, Moore DC: Anesthesiology 33:287, 1970
22. Boyes RN: Anesthésiques locaux en anesthésie et réanimation. Paris, Librairie Arnette, 1974, p 127

23. Foldes FF, Davidson GM, Duncalf D, Kuwabara S: Clin Pharmacol Ther 6:328, 1965
24. Åkerman B, Åström A, Ross S, Telĉ A: Acta Pharmacol Toxicol (Kbh) 24:389, 1966
25. Hjelm M, Holmdahl MH: Acta Anaesthesiol Scand 9:99, 1965
26. Brodie BB, Lief PA, Poet R: J Pharmacol Exp Ther 94:359, 1948
27. Sung CY, Truant AP: J Pharmacol Exp Ther 112:432, 1954
28. Hansson E, Hoffmann P, Kristerson L: Acta Pharmacol Toxicol (Kbh) 22:213, 1965
29. Foldes FF, Davis DL, Shanor S, Van Hees G: J Am Chem Soc 77:5149, 1955
30. Guidotti G: Arch Intern Med 129:194, 1972
31. Schmitt FO, Bear RS, Palmer KJ: J Cell Comp Physiol 18:31, 1941
32. Finean JB: Proceedings, 2nd International Conference, University of Ghent. London, Buttersworth, 1955, p 129
33. Robertson JD: Arch Intern Med 129:202, 1972
34. Danielli JF, Davson HA: J Cell Comp Physiol 9:89, 1936
35. Stein WD, Danielli JF: Discuss Faraday Soc 21:238, 1956
36. Robertson JD: Biochem Soc Symp 16:3, 1959
37. Lucy JA: J Theoret Biol 7:360, 1964
38. Green DW, Perdue JF: Proc Natl Acad Sci 55:1295, 1966
39. Benson AA: J Am Oil Chem Soc 43:265, 1966
40. Singer SJ, Nicolson GL: Science 175:720, 1972
41. Meymaris E: Br J Anaesthiol, (Suppl) 47:164, 1975
42. Camejo G, Villegas GM, Barnola FV, Villegas R: Biophys Acta 193:247, 1969
43. Boyes RN, Adams HJ, Covino BG: Rev Mex Anesth 23:81, 1974
44. Poppers PJ, Katz RL, Ericson EV, Meyer MB, Covino BG: Anesthesiology 40:13, 1974
45. Ling G, Gerard RW: J Cell Comp Physiol 34:383, 1949
46. Hodgkin AL: Biol Rev 26:339, 1951
47. Lechat P, Deleau D, Griffie RA: Med Exp (Basel) 11:157, 1964
48. Bromage PR, Burfoot MF: Br J Anaesthesiol 38:857, 1966
49. Aldrete JA, Barnes DR, Sidon MA, McMullen RB: Anesth Analg 48:269, 1969
50. Goldman D: J Gen Physiol 27:37, 1943
51. Hodgkin AL, Katz B: J Physiol 108:37, 1949
52. Hodgkin AL: Proc Roy Soc B 148:1, 1958
53. Shanes AM, Freygang WH, Grundfest H, Amatniek E: J Gen Physiol 42:793, 1959
54. Aceves J, Machne X: J Pharmacol Exp Ther 140:138, 1963
55. Condouris GA: J Pharmacol Exp Ther 131:243, 1961
56. Taylor RE: Am J Physiol 196:1071, 1959
57. Hille B: Nature 210:1220, 1966
58. Blaustein MP, Goldman DE: J Gen Physiol 49: 1043, 1966
59. Blaustein MP, Goldman DE: Science 153:429, 1966

60. Hille B: J Gen Physiol 51:199, 1968
61. Strichartz GR: J Gen Physiol 62:37, 1973
62. Hille B: J Gen Physiol 50:1287, 1967
63. Goldman DE, Blaustein MP: Ann NY Acad Sci 137:967, 1966
64. Bondani A, Karler R: J Cell Physiol 75:199, 1970
65. Papahadjopoulos D: Biochim Biophys Acta 211:467, 1970
66. Papahadjopoulos D: Biochim Biophys Acta 265:169, 1972
67. Kuperman AS, Altura BT, Chezar JA: Nature (Lond) 217:673, 1968
68. Grin J, Bueno EJ: Canadian J Physiol Pharmacol 51:516, 1973
69. Henderson R, Ritchie JM, Strichartz GR: J Physiol 235:783, 1973
70. Shanes AM: Pharmacol Rev 10:165, 1958
71. Ritchie JM, Ritchie B, Greengard P: J Pharmacol Exp Ther 150:152, 1965
72. Ritchie JM, Ritchie B, Greengard P: J Pharmacol Exp Ther 150:160, 1965
73. Dettbarn WD: Biochim Biophys Acta 57:73, 1962
74. Frazier DT, Narahashi T, Yamada M: J Pharmacol Exp Ther 171:45, 1970
75. Narahashi T, Yamada M, Frazier DT: Nature 223:748, 1969
76. Catchlove RFH: J Pharmacol Exp Ther 181:298, 1972
77. Condouris GA, Shakalis A: Nature 204:57, 1964
78. Catchlove RFH: Br J Anaesth 45:471, 1973
79. Bromage PR, Burfoot MF, Crowell DE, Truant AP: Br J Anaesth 39:197, 1967
80. Bromage PR: Acta Anaesth Scand, (Suppl) 16, p 55, 1965
81. Schülte-Steinberg O, Hartmuth J, Schutt L: Anaesthesia 25:191, 1970
82. de Jong, RH, Wagman IH: Anesthesiology 24:684, 1963
83. Ritchie JM, Greengard P: Ann Rev Pharmacol 6:405, 1966
84. Watson PJ: J Pharm Pharmacol 12:257, 1960
85. Kuperman AS, Okamato M, Beyer AM, Volpert WA: Science 144:1222, 1964
86. den Hertog A, Ritchie JM: Eur J Pharmacol 6:138, 1969
87. Feinstein MB, Paimre M: Biochim Biophys Acta 115:33, 1966
88. Åberg G: Acta Pharmacol Toxicol 31:273, 1972
89. Luduena FP, Bogado EF, Tullar BF: Arch Int Pharmacodyn Ther 200:359, 1972
90. Åkerman B: Doctoral dissertation. Uppsala, Sweden, 1973
91. Camougis G, Åkerman B, Sandberg R: Pharmacologist 9:205, 1967
92. Hille B, Courtney K, Dunn R: Molecular Mechanisms of Anesthesia. New York, Raven Press, 1975, p 13
93. Strichartz GR: J Gen Physiol 62:37, 1973
94. Narahashi T, Anderson NC, Moore JW: J Gen Physiol 50:1413, 1967
95. Zipf HR: Ger Med Meth 13:238, 1968
96. Ritchie JM: Br J Anaesth, (Suppl) 47, p 191, 1975
97. Ritchie JM, Ritchie BR: Science 162:1394, 1968
98. Skou JC: Acta Pharmacol Toxicol (Kbh) 10:281, 1954

99. Skou JC: Acta Pharmacol Toxicol (Kbh) 10:317, 1954
100. Skou JC: Acta Pharmacol Toxicol (Kbh) 10:325, 1954
101. Johnson SM, Miller K: Nature (Lond) 228:75, 1970
102. Seeman P: Pharmacol Rev 24:583, 1972
103. Takman B: Br J Anaesth, (Suppl) 47, p 183, 1975
104. Narahashi T, Frazier DT: Neurosci Rev 4:65, 1971
105. Mauro A, Truant AP, McCawley EL: Yale J Biol Med 21:113, 1948
106. Truant AP: Arch Int Pharmacodyn Ther 115:483, 1958
107. Camougis G, Takman BH: Methods Pharmacol 1:1, 1971
108. Meymaris E: Personal communication, 1975
109. Condouris GA, Shakalis A: Nature 204:57, 1964
110. Åström A, Persson NH: Br J Pharmacol 16:32, 1961
111. Heavner JE, de Jong RH: Personal communication, 1975
112. Colquhoun D, Ritchie JM: J Physiol 221:533, 1972
113. Colquhoun D, Ritchie JM: Mol Pharmacol 8:285, 1972
114. Covino BG: Anesthésiques Locaux en Anesthésie et Réanimation. Paris, Librairie Arnette, 1974, p 159
115. Covino BG: Adv Neurol 4:463, 1974
116. Luduena FP: Ann Rev Pharmacol 9:503, 1969
117. Bülbring E, Wajda I: J Pharmacol Exp Ther 85:78, 1945
118. Luduena FP, Hoppe JO: J Pharmacol Exp Ther 117:89, 1956
119. Wiedling S: Xylocaine: The Pharmacological Basis of its Clinical Use, ed 2. Stockholm, Almqvist and Wiksell, 1964
120. Duce BR, Zelechowski K, Camougis G, Smith ER: Br J Anaesth 41:579, 1969
121. Lebeaux M: Personal communication, 1975
122. Luduena FP: Arch Int Pharmacodyn Ther 109:143, 1957
123. Dvorak H, Manson MH: Proc Soc Exp Biol Med 28:344, 1930
124. Åström A, Persson NH: J Pharmacol Exp Ther 132:87, 1961
125. Adams HJ, Blair MR, Takman BH: Fed Proc 33:509, 1974
126. Åkerman B: Acta Pharmacol Toxicol 24:377, 1966
127. Defalque RJ, Stoelting VK: Anesth Analg 45:106, 1966
128. Covino BG, Bush DF: Br J Anaesth, (Suppl) 47, p 289, 1975
129. Swerdlow M, Jones R: Br J Anaesth 42:335, 1970
130. Evans CJ, Dewar JA, Boyes RN, Scott DB: Br J Anaesth 46:668, 1974
131. Bromage PR, Gertel M: Can Anaesth Soc J 17:557, 1970
132. Rubin AP, Lawson DIF: Anaesthesia 23:327, 1968
133. Fisher A, Bryce-Smith R: Anaesthesia 26:324, 1971
134. Szappanyos GG: Der Anaesthesist 18:330, 1969
135. Bromage PR: Br J Anaesth 34:161, 1962
136. Bromage PR, Gertel M: Anesthesiology 36:488, 1972
137. Eisele JH, Reitan JA: Anesthesiology 34:386, 1971
138. Lewis GBH: Can Anaesth Soc J 21:495, 1974
139. Quimby CW: Anesth Analg 44:387, 1965
140. Lund PC, Cwik JC, Gannon RT: Acta Anaesth Scand 18:176, 1974
141. Crawford OB: Anesthesiology 25:321, 1964

142. Albért J, Löfström B: Acta Anaesth Scand 9:203,1965
143. Scott DB, Jebson PJR, Braid DP, Örtengren B, Frisch P: Br J Anaesth 44:1040, 1972
144. Kier L: Acta Anaesth Scand 18:1, 1974
145. Bridenbaugh PO, Tucker GT, Moore DC, Bridenbaugh LD, Thompson GE, Balfour RI: Anesth Analg 53:430, 1974
146. Adriani J: Regional Anesthesia, ed 3. Philadelphia, W B Saunders, 1967
147. Gramling ZW, Ellis RG, Volpitto PP: J Med Assoc Ga 53:16, 1964
148. Padfield A: Anaesthesia 22:556, 1967
149. Ross NM, Dobbs EC: J Oral Surg: 21:215, 1963
150. Epstein S: J Am Dent Assoc 78:85, 1969
151. Björn H, Huldt S: Sven Tandlak Tidskr 40:831, 1947
152. Björn H: Sven Tandlak Tidskr (Suppl) 39, 1946
153. Cowan A: J Dent Res 43:1228, 1964
154. Bier A: Verh Dtsch Ges Chir 37:204, 1908
155. Bier A: Ann Surg 48:780, 1908
156. D'Amato H, Wiedling S (eds): Acta Anaesth Scand, (Suppl), 36, 1969
157. Thorn-Alquist AM: Acta Anaesth Scand, (Suppl) 40, p 7, 1971
158. Holmes CM: Lancet 1:245, 1963
159. Prevoznik SJ: Anesthesiology 32:177, 1970
160. Hargrove RL, Hoyle JR, Boyes RN, Beckett AH: Acta Anaesth Scand, (Suppl) 36, p 115, 1969
161. Mazze RI, Dunbar RW: Anesthesiology 27:574, 1966
162. Bell HM, Slater EM, Harris WH: JAMA 186:544, 1963
163. Atkinson DI, Modell J, Moya F: Anesth Analg 44:313, 1965
164. Kemmerer WT, Sampson ML, Heise DC: J Okla Med Assoc 59:221, 1966
165. Brown EM: Acta Anaesth Scand, (Suppl) 36, p 39, 1969
166. Harris WH, Slater EM, Bell HM: JAMA 194:1273, 1965
167. van Niekerk JP, Tonkin PA: S Afr Med J 40:165, 1966
168. Eriksson E, Persson A, Örtengren B: Acta Chir Scand, (Suppl) 358, p 47, 1966
169. Thorn-Alquist AM: Acta Anaesth Scand 13:229, 1969
170. Tucker GT, Boas RA: Anesthesiology 34:538, 1971
171. Cotev S, Robin GC: Acta Anaesth Scand, (Suppl) 36, p 127, 1969
172. Knapp RB, Weinberg M: JAMA 199:760, 1967
173. Adams JP, Dealy EJ, Kenmore PI: J Bone Joint Surg 46:811, 1964
174. de Jong RH, Nace RA: Anesthesiology 29:22, 1968
175. Miles DW, James JL, Clark DE: J Neurol Neurosurg Psychiatry 27:574, 1964
176. Shanks CA, McLeod JG: Br J Anaesth 42:1060, 1970
177. Sorbie C, Chacha P: Br Med J 1:957, 1965
178. Albért J, Löfström B: Acta Anaesth Scand 5:99, 1961
179. Albért J, Löfström B: Acta Anaesth Scand, (Suppl) 16, p 71, 1965
180. Albért J, Löfström B: Acta Anaesth Scand 9:1, 1965

181. Löfström B: Br J Anaesth, (Suppl) 47, p 297, 1975
182. Moore DC: Regional Block, ed 3. Springfield, Illinois, Charles C Thomas, 1961
183. Willdeck-Lund G, Edström H: Acta Anaesth Scand, (Suppl) 60, p 33, 1975
184. Moore DC, Bridenbaugh LD, Bridenbaugh PO, Tucker GT: Anesthesiology 32:78, 1970
185. Bridenbaugh PO, Moore DC, Bridenbaugh LD, Thompson GE: Acta Anaesthesia Scand 18:172, 1974
186. Winnie AP: Anesth Analg 49:455, 1970
187. Hollmen A, Mononen P: Acta Anaesth Scand, (Suppl) 60, p 25, 1975
188. Bromage PR, O'Biern P, Dunford LA: Can Anaesth Soc J 21:523, 1974
189. Tucker GT, Moore DC, Bridenbaugh PO, Bridenbaugh LD, Thompson GE: Anesthesiology 37:277, 1972
190. Bromage PR: Anesthesiology 28:592, 1967
191. Cheng PA: Anesth Analg 42:398, 1963
192. Shantha TR, Evans JA: Anesthesiology 37:543, 1972
193. Bromage PR: Br J Anaesth, (Suppl) 47, p 199, 1975
194. Bromage PR: Br J Anaesth 41:1016, 1969
195. Burn JM, Guyer PB, Langdon L: Br J Anaesth 45:338, 1973
196. Cohen EN: Anesthesiology 29:1002, 1968
197. Bromage PR, Joyal AC, Binney JC: Science 140:392, 1963
198. Urban BJ: Anesthesiology 39:496, 1973
199. Galindo A, Hernandez J, Benavides O, Ortegon de Muñoz S, Bonica JJ: Br J Anaesth 47:41, 1975
200. Lund PC, Bush D, Covino BG: Anesthesiology 42:497, 1975
201. Erdemir HA, Soper LE, Sweet RB: Anesth Analg 44:400, 1965
202. Nishimura N, Kitahara T, Kusakabe T: Anesthesiology 20:785, 1959
203. Hehre FW, Moyes AZ, Senfield RM, Lilly EJ: Anesth Analg 44:89, 1965
204. Hehre FW, Yules RB, Hipona FA: Anesth Analg 945:551, 1966
205. Lund PC: Peridural Analgesia and Anesthesia. Springfield, Illinois, Charles C Thomas, 1966
206. Waters HR, Rosen N, Perkins DH: Anaesthesia 25:184, 1970
207. Watt MJ, Akhtar M, Atkinson RS: Anaesthesia 25:24, 1970
208. Lund PC, Cwik JC, Vallesteros F: Anesth Analg 49:103, 1970
209. Moore DC, Bridenbaugh LD, Bridenbaugh PO, Tucker GT: JAMA 214:713, 1970
210. Engberg G, Holmdahl M, Edstrom HH: Acta Anaesth Scand 18:277, 1974
211. Stanton-Hicks M, Murphy TM, Bonica JJ, Berges PU, Mather LE, Tucker GT: Anesthesiology 42:398, 1975
212. Braid DP, Scott DB: Br J Anaesth 37:394, 1965
213. Thorn-Alquist AM, Edström H: Acta Anaesth Scand, (Suppl) 60, p 64, 1975
214. Stanton-Hicks M, Berges PU, Bonica JJ: Anesthesiology 39:308, 1973

215. Erlanger J, Gasser HS: Am J Physiol 70:624, 1924
216. Daos FG, Virtue RW: JAMA 183:285, 1963
217. Dripps RD, Vandam LD: JAMA 156:1486, 1954
218. Moore DC, Bridenbaugh LD: JAMA 195:907, 1966
219. Phillips OC, Ebner H, Nelson AT, Black MH: Anesthesiology 30:284, 1969
220. Bergmann H: Der Anaesthesist 21:133, 1972
221. Noble AB, Murray JG: Can Anaesth Soc J 18:5, 1971
222. Moore DC, Bridenbaugh LD, Bagdi PA, Bridenbaugh PO, Stander H: Anesth Analg 47:40, 1968
223. Mörch ET, Rosenberg MK, Truant AT: Acta Anaesth Scand 1:105, 1957
224. Sadove MS, Sanchez JD: J Int Col Surg 39:45, 1963
225. Neigh JL, Kane PB, Smith TC: Anesth Analg 49:912, 1970
226. Lund PC: Principles and Practice of Spinal Anesthesia. Springfield, Illinois, Charles C Thomas, 1971
227. Barclay DL, Reneger OJ, Nelson EW: Am J Obstet Gynecol 101:792, 1968
228. Kallos T, Smith TC: Anesth Analg 51:766, 1972
229. Louthan BW, Jones JR, Henschel EO, Jacoby J: Anesth Analg 44:742, 1965
230. Crispell R: J Am Osteopath Assoc 69:578, 1970
231. Meagher RP, Moore DC, Devries JC: Anesth Analg 45:134, 1966
232. Smith SM, Ree VL: Anesthesiology 9:229, 1948
233. Bromage PR, Pettigrew RT, Crowell DE: J Clin Pharmacol 9:30, 1969
234. Cohen EN, Levine DA, Colliss JE, Gunther RE: Anesthesiology 29:994, 1968
235. Covino BG: N Engl J Med 286:975, 1035, 1972
236. Proctor DG: Anesthesiology 29:1025, 1968
237. Thorton JA, Johnston J: Anaesthesia 19:576, 1964
238. Purnell RJ, Frew RM, Roth IZ: Anaesthesia 21:480, 1966
239. Polk JW, Bailey AH: Dis Chest 51:293, 1967
240. Jankelson IR, Jankelson OM: Am J Gastroenterol 32:636, 1959
241. Hollander E: Am J Gastroenterol 34:613, 1960
242. Seifter J, Glassman JM, Hudyma GM: Proc Soc Exp Biol Med 109:664, 1962
243. Rheault MJ, Semb LS, Harkins HN, Nyhus LM: Am J Dig Dis 10:128, 1965
244. Langston JB, Yeager PA, Simrell WD, Hogg M: Invest Urol 5:149, 1967
245. Adriani J: Clin Pharmacol Ther 1:645, 1960
246. Adriani J, Zepernick R, Arens J, Authement E: Clin Pharmacol Ther 5:49, 1964
247. Adriani J, Zepernick R: JAMA 188:93, 1964
248. Adriani J, Zepernick R: Ann Surg 158:666, 1963

249. Adriani J, Dalili H: Anesth Analg 50:834, 1971
250. Lubens HM, Ausdenmoore RW, Shafer AD, Reece RM: Am J Dis Child 128:192, 1974
251. Giddon DB, Quadland M, Rachwall PC, Springer J, Tursky B: J Oral Ther Pharmacol 4:270, 1968
252. Schwartz ML, Covino BG, Narang RM, Sethi V, Tholpady SS, Kuangparichat M, et al: Am Heart J 88:721; 1974
253. DiGiovanni AJ: Anesthesiology 34:92, 1971
254. Meyer MB, Zelechowski K: Lidocaine in the Treatment of Ventricular Arrhythmias. Edinburgh, E & S Livingstone, p 161, 1971
255. Cohen LS, Rosenthal JE, Horner DW, Atkins JM, Matthews OA, Sarnoff S: Am J Cardiol 29:520, 1972
256. Schwartz ML, Meyer MB, Covino BG, Narang RM, Sethi V, Schwartz AJ, et al: J Clin Pharmacol 14:77, 1974
257. Evans EF, Proctor JD, Fratkin MJ, Velandia J, Wasserman AJ: Clin Pharmacol Ther 17:44, 1975
258. Boyes RN, Adams HJ, Duce BR: J Pharmacol Exp Ther 174:1, 1970
259. Boyes RN, Scott DB, Jebson PJ, Godman MJ, Julian DG: Clin Pharmacol Ther 12:105, 1971
260. Adriani J, Campbell D: JAMA 162:1527, 1956
261. Eriksson E, Englesson S, Wahlqvist S, Örtengren B: Acta Chir Scand, (Suppl) 358, p 25, 1966
262. Lund PC, Covino BG: J Clin Pharmacol 7:324, 1967
263. Blair MR: Br J Anaesth, (Suppl) 47, p 247, 1975
264. Dhunér K-G, Lewis DH: Acta Anaesth Scand, (Suppl) 23, p 347, 1966
265. Scott DB, Jebson PJR, Boyes RN: Br J Anaesth 45:1010, 1973
266. Nishimura N, Morioka T, Sato S, Kuba T: Anesth Analg 44:135, 1965
267. MacMillan WH: Br J Pharmacol 14:385, 1959
268. Tucker GT, Mather LE: Br J Anaesth, (Suppl) 47, p 213, 1975
269. de Jong RH, Heavner JE, de Oliveira L: Anesthesiology 37:493, 1972
270. Katz J: Anesthesiology 29:249, 1968
271. Kristerson L, Hoffmann P, Hansson E: Acta Pharmacol Toxicol 22:205, 1965
272. Sjöstrand U, Widman B: Acta Anaesth Scand, (Suppl) 50, p 24, 1973
273. Rowland M, Thomson PD, Guichard A, Melmon KL: Ann NY Acad Sci 179:383, 1971
274. Thomson PD, Melmon KL, Richardson JA, Cohn K, Steinbrunn W, Cudihee R, et al: Ann Intern Med 78:499, 1973
275. Morishima HO, Daniel SS, Finster M, Poppers P, James LS: Anesthesiology 27:147, 1966
276. Thomas J, Climie CR, Mather LE: Br J Anaesth 40:965, 1968
277. Shnider SM, Way EL: Anesthesiology 29:944, 1968
278. Shnider SM, Way EL: Anesthesiology 29:951, 1968
279. Epstein BS, Banerjee SG, Coakley CS: Anesth Analg 47:223, 1968
280. Moore DC, Bridenbaugh LD, Bagdi PA, Bridenbaugh PO: Anesthesiology 29:585, 1968

281. Poppers PJ, Finster M: Anesthesiology 29:1134, 1968
282. Thomas J, Climie CR, Mather LE: Br J Anaesth 41:1035, 1969
283. Fox GS, Houle GL: Can Anaesth Soc J 16:135, 1969
284. Hehre FW, Hook R, Hon EH: Anesth Analg 48:909, 1969
285. Reynolds F, Taylor G: Anaesthesia 25:14, 1970
286. Poppers PJ: Br J Anaesth, (Suppl) 47, p 322, 1975
287. Covino BG: Anesthesiology 35:158, 1971
288. Finster M, Morishima HO, Boyes RN, Covino BG: Anesthesiology 36:159, 1972
289. Finster M: Personal communication, 1975
290. Tucker GT, Boyes RN, Bridenbaugh PO, Moore DC: Anesthesiology 33:303, 1970
291. Mather LE, Long G, Thomas J: J Pharm Pharmacol 23:359, 1971
292. Foldes FF, Foldes VM, Smith JC, Zsigmond EK: Anesthesiology 24:208, 1963
293. Geddes IC: Acta Anaesth Scand, (Suppl) 16, p 37, 1965
294. Keenaghan JB: Personal communication, 1975
295. Aldrete JA, Homatas J, Boyes RN, Starzl TE: Anesth Analg 49:687, 1970
296. Stenson RE, Constantino RT, Harrison DC: Circulation 43:205, 1971
297. Selden R, Sasahara AA: JAMA 202:908, 1967
298. Boyes RN: Br J Anaesth, (Suppl) 47, p 225, 1975
299. Hollunger G: Acta Pharmacol Toxicol 17:365, 1960
300. Keenaghan JB, Boyes RN: J Pharmacol Exp Therap 180:454, 1972
301. Breck GD, Trager WF: Science 173:544, 1971
302. Mather LE, Thomas J: Life Sci 11:915, 1972
303. Nelson SD, Breck GD, Trager WF: J Med Chem 16:1106, 1973
304. Nelson SD, Garland WA, Trager WF: Res Commun Chem Pathol Pharmacol 8:45, 1974
305. Thomas J, Meffin P: J Med Chem 15:1046, 1972
306. Meffin P, Robertson AV, Thomas J, Winkler J: Xenobiotica 3:191, 1973
307. Meffin P, Thomas J: Xenobiotica 3:625, 1973
308. Meffin P, Long GJ, Thomas J: Clin Pharmacol Ther 14:218, 1973
309. Reynolds F: Br J Anaesth 43:567, 1971
310. Goehl TJ, Davenport JB, Stanley MJ: Xenobiotica 3:761, 1973
311. Smith ER, Duce BR: J Pharmacol Exp Ther 179:580, 1971
312. Strong JM, Parker M, Atkinson AJ: Clin Pharmacol Ther 14:67, 1973
313. Beckett AH, Boyes RN, Appleton PJ: J Pharm Pharmacol 18:76S, 1966
314. Eriksson E, Granberg P-O: Acta Anaesth Scand, (Suppl) 16, p 79, 1965
315. Ryrfeldt A, Hansson E: Acta Pharmacol Toxicol 30:59, 1971
316. Eriksson E, Persson A: Acta Chir Scand, (Suppl) 358, p 37, 1966
317. Usubiaga JE, Wikinski J, Ferrero R, Usubiaga LE, Wikinski R: Anesth Analg 45:611, 1966
318. Scott DB: Br J Anaesth 47:56, 1975

319. Wagman IH, de Jong RH, Prince DA: Anesthesiology 28:155, 1967
320. Tanaka K, Yamasaki M: Nature 209:207, 1966
321. de Jong RH, Robles R, Corbin RW: Anesthesiology 30:19, 1969
322. Huffman RD, Yim GKW: Int J Neuropharmacology 8:217, 1969
323. Warnick JE, Kee RD, Yim GKW: Anesthesiology 34:327, 1971
324. Åström A, Persson NH, Örtengren B: Acta Pharmacol Toxicol 21:161, 1964
325. Munson ES, Gutnick MJ, Wagman IH: Anesth Analg 49:986, 1970
326. Munson ES, Martucci RW, Wagman IH: Br J Anaesth 44:1025, 1972
327. Englesson S: Doctoral thesis, University of Uppsala, Sweden, 1973
328. Munson ES, Tucker WK, Ansinsch B, Malagodi MH: Anesthesiology 42:471, 1975
329. de Jong RH, Wagman IH, Prince DA: Exp Neurol 17:221, 1967
330. Munson ES, Wagman IH: Arch Neurol 20:406, 1969
331. Sakabe T, Maekawa T, Ishikawa T, Takeshita H: Anesthesiology 40:433, 1974
332. de Jong RH, Heavner JE: Anesthesiology 34:523, 1971
333. de Jong RH, Heavner JE, de Oliveira LF: Exp Neurol 35:558, 1972
334. de Jong RH, Heavner JE, de Oliveira LF: Anesthesiology 37:299, 1972
335. de Jong RH, Heavner JE: Can Anaesth Soc J 21:153, 1974
336. Aldrete JA, Daniel W: Anesth Analg 50:127, 1971
337. Richards RK, Smith NT, Katz J: Anesthesiology 29:493, 1968
338. de Jong RH, Heavner JE: Anesthesiology 36:449, 1972
339. Munson ES, Wagman IH: Anesthesiology 37:523, 1972
340. Munson ES, Wagman IH: Arch Neurol 28:329, 1973
341. Bernhard CG, Bohm E: Local Anaesthetics as Anticonvulsants. Stockholm, Almqvist and Wiksell, 1965
342. Julien RM, Demetrescu M: J Life Sci 4:27, 1974
343. Demetrescu M, Julien RM: Epilepsia 15:235, 1974
344. Julien RM: Electroencephalogr Clin Neurophysiol 34:639, 1973
345. Essman WB: Arch Int Pharmacodyn 164:376, 1966
346. Essman WB: Arch Int Pharmacodyn 157:166, 1965
347. Essman WB: Arch Int Pharmacodyn 171:159, 1968
348. Wikinski JA, Usubiaga JE, Morales RL, Torrieri A, Usubiaga LE: Anesth Analg 49:504, 1970
349. Davis LD, Temte JV: Circ Res 24:639, 1969
350. Bigger JT, Mandel WJ: J Clin Invest 49:63, 1970
351. Bigger JT, Mandel WJ: J Pharmacol Exp Ther 172:239, 1970
352. Harrison DC, Sprouse JH, Morrow AG: Circulation 28:486, 1963
353. Lieberman NA, Harris RS, Katz RI: Am J Cardiol 22:375, 1968
354. Sugimoto T, Schaal SF, Dunn NM, Wallace AG: J Pharmacol Exp Ther 166:146, 1969
355. Rosen KM, Lau SH, Weiss MB, Damato AN: Am J Cardiol 25:1, 1970
356. Kabela E: J Pharmacol Exp Ther 184:611, 1973

357. Dunbar RW, Boettner RB, Gatz RN, Pennington RE, Morrow DH: Anesth Analg 49:761, 1970
358. Katz RL: Acta Anaesth Scand, (Suppl) 16, p 29, 1965
359. Austen WG, Moran JM: Am J Cardiol 16:701, 1965
360. Kao FF, Jalar UH: Br J Pharmacol 14:522, 1959
361. Stewart DM, Rogers WP, Mahaffey JE, Witherspoon S, Woods EF: Anesthesiology 24:620, 1963
362. Nayler WG, McInnes I, Carson V, Stone J, Lowe TE: Am Heart J 78:338, 1969
363. Jewitt DE, Kishon Y, Thomas M: Lancet 1:266, 1968
364. Stannard M, Sloman G, Sangster L: Br Med J 2:468, 1968
365. Schumacher RR, Lieberson AD, Childress RH, Williams JF: Circulation 37:965, 1968
366. Klein SW, Sutherland RIL, Morch JE: Can Med Assoc J 99:472, 1968
367. Binnion PF, Murtagh G, Pollock AM, Fletcher E: Br Med J 3:390, 1969
368. Grossman JI, Cooper JA, Frieden J: Am J Cardiol 24:191, 1969
369. Åström A: Acta Physiol Scand 60:30, 1964
370. Sanders HD: Can J Physiol Pharmacol 49:218, 1969
371. Åberg G, Wahlstrom B: Acta Pharmacol Toxicol 31:255, 1972
372. Jörfeldt L, Löfström B, Pernow B, Wahren J: Acta Anaesthesiol Scand 14:183, 1970
373. Sanders HD: Can J Physiol Pharmacol 43:39, 1965
374. Åberg G, Dhunér K-G: Acta Pharmacol Toxicol 31:267, 1972
375. Åberg G, Mörck E, Waldeck B: Acta Pharmacol Toxicol 33:476, 1973
376. Åberg G, Andersson R: Acta Pharmacol Toxicol 31:321, 1972
377. Somlyo AP, Somlyo AV: Pharmacol Rev 22:2, 1970
378. McWhirter W, Frederickson E, Steinhaus J: South Med J 65:796, 1972
379. McWhirter W, Schmidt FH, Frederickson E, Steinhaus J: Anesthesiology 39:398, 1973
380. de Jong RH, Heavner JE: Anesthesiology 39:633, 1973
381. Bromage PR: Anaesthesia 6:26, 1951
382. Bonica JJ, Backup PH, Anderson CE, Hadfield D, Crepps WF, Monk BF: Anesthesiology 18:723, 1957
383. Defalque RJ: Anesthesiology 23:627, 1962
384. Ward RJ, Bonica JJ, Freund FG, Akamatsu TJ, Danziger F, Englesson S: JAMA 191:275, 1965
385. Stanton-Hicks M: Br J Anaesth, (Suppl) 47, p 253, 1975
386. Bonica JJ, Berges PU, Morikawa K: Anesthesiology 33:619, 1970
387. Kennedy WF, Sawyer TK, Gerbershagen HV, Cutter RE, Allen GD, Bonica JJ: Anesthesiology 31:414, 1969
388. Kennedy WF, Everett GB, Cobb LA, Allen GD: Anesth Analg 50:1069, 1971
389. Bonica JJ, Akamatsu TJ, Berges PU, Morikawa K, Kennedy WF: Anesthesiology 34:514, 1971

390. Bonica JJ, Kennedy WF, Akamatsu TJ, Gerbershagen HU: Anesthesiology 36:219, 1972
391. Martin WE, Everett G, Kennedy WF, Allen G: Anesth Analg 52:454, 1973
392. Weiss EG: Personal communication, 1974
393. Jörfeldt L, Löfström B, Pernow B, Persson B, Wahren J, Widman B: Acta Anaesth Scand 12:153, 1968
394. Sjögren S, Wright B: Acta Anaesth Scand 16:27, 1972
395. Wahba WM, Craig DB, Don HF, Becklake MR: Can Anaesth Soc J 19:8, 1972
396. Spence AA, Smith G: Br J Anaesth 43:144, 1971
397. Hollmén A, Saukkonen J: Acta Anaesth Scand 16:147, 1972
398. Hollmén A, Korhonen M, Ojala A: Br J Anaesth 41:603, 1969
399. Hollmén A, Ojala A, Korhonen M: Acta Anaesth Scand 13:1, 1969
400. Sinha YK: J Pharm Pharmacol 5:620, 1953
401. Katz RL, Gissen AJ: Acta Anaesth Scand, (Suppl) 36, p 103, 1969
402. Wiedling S: Acta Pharmacol Toxicol 17:233, 1960
403. Wiedling S: Xylocaine®: The Pharmacological Basis of its Clinical Use. Stockholm, Almqvist and Wiksell, 1959
404. Schmidt RM, Rosenkranz HS: J Infect Dis 121:597, 1970
405. Hirst GDS, Wood DR: Br J Pharmacol 41:94, 1971
406. Hirst GDS, Wood DR: Br J Pharmacol 41:105, 1971
407. Galindo A: J Pharmacol Exp Ther 177:360, 1971
408. Telivuo L: Acta Anaesth Scand 11:327, 1967
409. Deguchi T, Narahashi T: J Pharmacol Exp Ther 176:423, 1971
410. Ghoneim MM: Can Anaesth Soc J 18:353, 1971
411. DeKornfeld TJ, Steinhaus JE: Anesth Analg 38:173, 1959
412. Hall DR, McGibbon DH, Evans CC, Meadows GA: Br J Anaesth 44:1329, 1972
413. Heinonen J: Acta Pharmacol 21:155, 1964
414. Smudski JW, Sprecher RL, Elliott HW: Arch Oral Biol 9:595, 1964
415. Heinonen J, Takki S, Jarho L: Acta Anaesth Scand 14:89, 1970
416. DiFazio CA, Brown RE: Anesthesiology 36:238, 1972
417. Bonica JJ: Clinical Applications of Diagnostic and Therapeutic Nerve Blocks. Springfield, Illinois, Charles C Thomas, 1959
418. Collins VJ: Principles of Anesthesiology. Philadelphia, Lea & Febiger, 1966
419. Ross NM: Anesth Progr 13:139, 1966
420. Waldman HB, Binkley G: J Am Dent Assoc 74:747, 1967
421. Holti G, Hood FJC: Dent Pract Dent Res 15:294, 1965
422. Aldrete JA, Johnson DA: Anesth Analg 49:173, 1970
423. Aldrete JA, Johnson DA: JAMA 207:356, 1969
424. Dawkins CJM: Anaesthesia 24:554, 1969
425. Skou JC: Acta Pharmacol Toxicol (Kbh) 10:292, 1954
426. Giddon DB, Lindhe J: Am J Pathol 68:327, 1972
427. Benoit PW, Belt WD: J Anat 107:547, 1970

428. Benoit PW, Belt WD: Exp Neurol 34:264, 1972
429. Adams HJ, Mastri AR, Eicholzer A, Kilpatrick G: Anesth Analg 53:904, 1974
430. Fink BR, Kennedy RD, Hendrickson AE, Middaugh ME: Anesthesiology 36:422, 1972
431. MacDonald AD, Watkins KH: Br J Surg 25:879, 1938
432. Adams HJ, Mastri A: Personal communication, 1974
433. Libelius R, Sonesson B, Stamenović BA, Thesleff S: J Anat 106:297, 1970
434. Zener JC, Harrison DC: Arch Int Med 134:48, 1974
435. Lund PC: Acta Anaesth Scand 6:143, 1962

Index